The International Library

MODERN PSYCHOLOGY AND EDUCATION

Founded by C. K. Ogden

The International Library of Psychology

DEVELOPMENTAL PSYCHOLOGY
In 32 Volumes

MODERN PSYCHOLOGY AND EDUCATION

A Text-Book of Psychology for Students in Training Colleges and Adult Evening Classes

MARY STURT AND E C OAKDEN

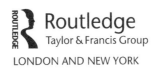

Routledge
Taylor & Francis Group
LONDON AND NEW YORK

First published in 1926 by
Kegan Paul, Trench, Trubner & Co., Ltd.
2 Park Square, Milton Park, Abingdon, Oxfordshire OX14 4RN
711 Third Avenue, New York, NY 10017

First issued in paperback 2014

Routledge is an imprint of the Taylor and Francis Group, an informa business

© 1926 Mary Sturt and E C Oakden

All rights reserved. No part of this book may be reprinted or reproduced
or utilized in any form or by any electronic, mechanical, or other means,
now known or hereafter invented, including photocopying
and recording, or in any information storage or retrieval system, without
permission in writing from the publishers.

The publishers have made every effort to contact authors/copyright holders
of the works reprinted in the *International Library of Psychology*.
This has not been possible in every case, however, and we would
welcome correspondence from those individuals/companies
we have been unable to trace.

These reprints are taken from original copies of each book. In many cases
the condition of these originals is not perfect. The publisher has gone to
great lengths to ensure the quality of these reprints, but wishes to point
out that certain characteristics of the original copies will, of necessity, be
apparent in reprints thereof.

British Library Cataloguing in Publication Data
A CIP catalogue record for this book
is available from the British Library

Modern Psychology and Education
ISBN 0415-21009-7
Developmental Psychology: 32 Volumes
ISBN 0415-21128-X
The International Library of Psychology: 204 Volumes
ISBN 0415-19132-7

ISBN 13: 978-1-138-87517-3 (pbk)
ISBN 13: 978-0-415-21009-6 (hbk)

" Alack, poor soul, thou hast need of more rags to lay on thee, rather than have these off."

CONTENTS

vii

CONTENTS

PREFACE

THE aim of this book is to put before students beginning psychology a sketch of the subject which may be comprehensible to them because it deals with common experience illustrated by concrete cases. These examples are not drawn from a doctor's practice, but are in a large part records of events such as take place every day. In addition to this there are frequent references to literature, since the psychological knowledge of an age is largely enshrined in its fiction, poetry, and drama.

Two classes of students have been kept specially in mind throughout :

(1) Evening-class students, of the type who attend W.E.A. lectures, and who wish to gain a general insight into their own minds and those of others ;

(2) Students in training colleges, who need their psychology for a definite examination as well as for general culture. These students might use this book as a three-term course. It covers the psychological part of an ordinary education syllabus, and should enable students to answer the psychological questions in a Principles of Education paper.

The book has also another aim in relation to these students. It is hoped that it may enable them to sympathize somewhat more with the children they are going to teach, and also to adapt themselves more rapidly to the demands of school life.

Behind this lies another plea. Educational psychology in the past has been almost exclusively the psychology of the child, and the psychology of the teacher has been neglected. Yet the teacher is one half of the teaching situation, and, unless conditions are so arranged that the teacher can develop his maximum efficiency, the children

ix

are bound to suffer. The teacher often works under conditions which would not be tolerated for a moment in any well-organized factory. Secondary and elementary schools are alike culpable, though frequently in different ways.

In going round the elementary schools in some districts, no impartial person could fail to be struck by the extremely bad conditions under which many of the teachers work. The buildings are old, badly ventilated, and so generally grimy that no effort on a teacher's part will make the room attractive. Frequently the teachers have no proper staff-room, and the corner they have is insufficiently provided with chairs. The sanitary conditions are often shocking, and there is no water in the tap to enable anybody to wash. In the country they may come from a distance and eat their lunch in school without such arrangements as would make the food reasonably palatable. In towns the school buildings are in such noisy places that during much of a lesson the teacher cannot be heard. In general, the teacher spends each day from 8.45 till 4.45 in a continual state of bustle, noise and strain, and all but the strongest rapidly show the effects.

The proportion of badly equipped secondary schools is smaller, but on the whole (except for the greater length of holiday) the conditions for the teachers are worse. The hours of work in school are approximately the same (8.45 to 4.15 or 4.45), and the lunch interval is frequently occupied by school tasks of various kinds, whilst the staff-room is generally too small to allow of any real repose. But it is out of school that these teachers' task is so much heavier. Suppose that in a school of three hundred children a teacher takes one subject throughout the school, she will be expected to set written work about twice a week to each class, and will therefore have six hundred exercises to correct in the course of the week, i.e. a hundred each evening. In addition to this correcting she will have to prepare six or seven lessons a day, some of them involving advanced work. No one can correct more than sixty books in an hour, so that corrections take at least two hours, and the preparation of lessons probably one more. The total day's work is, therefore, ten hours at least.

PREFACE

A student leaving college is cast into this life with no real preparation or explanation. His headmaster, having been through it himself, too often thinks that it is all for the best, and makes no effort to help, but rather sees in the young teacher's misery an opportunity for enforcing his own ideas and methods ; with the result that another teacher is produced of the type held up to ridicule in so many novels. At various points through this book hints have been given which it is trusted may be of help to those who are about to face this situation.

What is really needed is a new educational psychology which is concerned with the teacher. Of late years in England an Industrial Psychology has sprung up which attempts to study working conditions in the joint interest of workers and employers. Investigators have been trained and a technique developed. As every year passes the value of this work becomes more obvious. Not only do experts study the material and mental conditions of work, they also advise as to which people are most fitted for special types of work.

The teaching profession needs an investigation on these lines. An enormous part of the strain and misery of a teacher's life is directly due to stupidity, bad organization and meanness. If the National Union of Teachers, or some organization of secondary-school teachers, would insist on an investigation of their conditions of work, circulate a report, and do their best to get it acted on, a new era might open for teachers and consequently for education in England and the world.

INTRODUCTION

THE SCOPE OF THE BOOK

" What a piece of work is man ! "

IT is never easy to write a text-book, and psychology is a subject which presents exceptional difficulties. The word itself claims that psychology is the study of the soul of man, but as we can only study the soul through its manifestations, all the works of man, from one point of view, come legitimately within the limits of the subject. To take an example, a cathedral represents an idea in the minds of the builders, and we can learn much of the thoughts of the age in which it was built from the study of it. To the psychologist, therefore, a cathedral is relevant material, though the mechanics of the building and the strains of the masonry are irrelevant. History is one long record of the minds of men in action ; a large part of literature is nothing but careful studies of character thrown into a fictitious form, but deriving their value from their connection with real life. The psychologist may well say :

" Homo sum ; humani nihil a me alienum puto."

The very richness of his field embarrasses him. Not only does he study the mind of man as displayed in history or concrete achievements, but he observes the behaviour of the living human beings with whom he comes into daily contact ; he goes farther and compares the behaviour of his cat or dog, of monkeys, of amœbæ, with that of man, and, from this comparison, he hopes to understand better the behaviour of the people about him.

As is natural, no one psychologist ever hopes to cover the whole of this vast field. Inevitably one must confine oneself to some particular point, and can only refer to other branches or draw an occasional illustration from them. This book will confine itself to the workings of the mind as we can observe it in ourselves or in our immediate neighbours, and when other topics are treated they will be introduced simply for the purpose of making human impulses and actions more explicable.

In consequence, vast stretches of the subject will be completely omitted, and others dismissed with a brief reference. In the opinion of the writers the sections chosen are the most interesting and the most important, especially for those people who have to deal continually with numbers of their fellow men ; but the student must not for one moment imagine that more than the smallest fraction of all the interesting things which might be said on this subject are contained in this book, or that, however far he chooses to roam, he will come up against a dead wall of dogma precluding all farther speculation.

Nothing is so infinite in its variations as the human mind ; and each explorer, having one of his own, is in as good a position for study as any other investigator. In some subjects there are " laws of nature " which demand acceptance ; in psychology anyone who studies the question carefully has a right to his own opinion, and in no subject is dogmatism, or intolerance of a contrary opinion more out of place. It is hoped that anyone who reads this book will test each point in it by his own experience, and decline to accept what he feels he can reasonably well disprove.

There is another difficulty inherent in writing a psychological text-book, apart from the breadth of the subject, and that is the metaphysical questions which are always being suggested, and to which psychology has little answer to give.

We said above that the word " psychology " means the study of the soul. But what is the soul ? How is it connected with the mind and the body ? Are we to think of the spiritual part of our being in a manner suggested by Dante and mediæval church paintings, as going to heaven in a white shirt if we are good, or to hell naked if we are bad ? Is the mind, our power of thought, merely a tool of the soul ?—or is mind the highest function of the soul, as Plato and Aristotle say ? Or, again, have we one unitary soul, or is our non-material being, like our physical frame, built up of many component parts ; and if the soul is composite, how can a non-material thing (supposing the soul is non-material) have *parts*, and what relation can these parts bear to each other ?

Then, again, to ourselves we seem to know our own existence and to perceive the world about us. What is this knowledge of ourselves, this consciousness, and how exactly, in this respect, do we differ from a stone which we believe lacks this consciousness ? We are alive and the stone is dead. Yes, but what does being alive mean, except the liability to death ? And are we not dust, waiting to return to dust again ?

The world about us looks distinct and real enough, but so do the landscapes of our dreams. What *is* reality and how do we get into touch with it ? We claim that a thing is real if it fits into a scheme of probability, if water flows downhill and " the sparks fly upward " ; yet at any moment a new fact may break through our net of reason and condemn our world, or itself, to unreality.

It is all very difficult ; but, fortunately, it is outside the direct province of psychology. The metaphysicians themselves are fair game, and it is, to say the least, an amusing and legitimate pursuit to try to deduce the mental peculiarities which led Plato to form the theory of ideas, and Hegel to declare that " true freedom is conformity to law ". It is also good for us to walk up to the edge of the gulf and look over. Holding our own soul firmly by the hand and refusing for a minute to doubt its existence, it is pleasant to watch the metaphysicians plunging into the waves of doubt and scepticism. It is even good sometimes to turn to our own soul and say : " Are you really there, old fellow, one and the same ? or are you constructed like an onion, ring on ring and layer on layer ? " It really does not matter what answer we get. It is interesting to have asked the question. So, too, now and then, we do well to doubt the reality of the world ; to feel that " nothing is but what is not ", and decide that all is " vanity ". This denial of the importance of the phenomenal world lies at the basis

3

of Buddhist teaching, and has been the refuge of many who have been wearied by conflict with the world.

If psychology does not feel called upon to deal with these questions it is because to ordinary perception there seems little doubt about them. There is the old argument employed against the idealist metaphysician ; when he hits his toe against a stone, does he still believe in the unreality of matter ? We can study our perceptions of things, but *things* they remain for us though we learn that they are certainly not as we perceive them. So, too, we can get to know more about our mind or soul and its composition, yet we do not lose the conviction with which we started ; that it is there, a personal entity. It will be useless, therefore, to look in this book for the discussion of such questions. A certain number of references will be given to books where they are discussed, and those readers who have a taste for such fascinating speculations may find them there.

The difficulties of psychology in part account for its interest, but the greatest appeal that it makes is to our egoism. Psychology is a study of ourselves, and we all enjoy that. Even explaining our symptoms to a doctor gives us a certain pleasure, and our minds are more intimate and interesting than our bodies. Moreover, it puts our neighbours in a new light. Jones ceases to be that " irritating self-assertive bore ", and becomes a peculiarly instructive case of a " inferiority complex ". We may even seek Jones's society now and try to discover his previous history and the " ætiology of his symptoms ".

Further, with the resources psychology opens to us, we need never be dull ; for if we are, we can start analysing our own state of mind, and attempt to formulate the exact mental processes which go on in the different stages of boredom. It is even possible to find a scientific interest in more unpleasant events, for, with a little practice, we can learn to look at ourselves from without, and thus, adopting the attitude of a spectator, decrease our own immediate sense of misery, and diminish the overwhelming importance of our personal sorrows.

It is for this among other reasons that psychology should be taught. It is a very good hobby, and will lend zest to our reading and to our observation of people and places, but it has a use beyond that. If the study is successful it should bring to the student a greater power of self-criticism and a greater tolerance of others. To understand all is to pardon all, and, though one may be far from completely understanding a given case, the general attitude of mind of one who seeks humbly for reasons for conduct is more helpful and desirable in society than the attitude of one who observes closely only to criticize, to judge and to approve or condemn.

But, although the study of psychology serves a moral end, it is not in itself concerned with morals—except in so far as it takes cognizance of the state of mind of those who hold or invent them. Actions, from a psychological point of view, are not " right " and " wrong ". They may be socially desirable or the reverse, or indicative of health or disease. Psychology registers the fact that these states of mind exist and seeks to explain them, not to pass judgment on them. A very little thought shows that any system of morals is relative to particular circumstances of place and time. A scientist who is concerned in trying to discover permanent elements in human conduct is not concerned to judge the actions which spring from these elements in terms of the morality current at his own day, any more than he would judge them in terms of that current in 1000 B.C.

We must not, however, from this conclude that psychology is merely a matter of knowledge and pleasantly divorced from practice. Psychology may be described as the art of getting one's own way. The teacher who studies it does so mainly to learn how to control and teach his class with the least trouble to himself and the greatest profit to them. The modern politician studies methods of propaganda for the purpose of governing a united nation. The youngest child knows how to control his family, and any intelligent dog knows the best methods of getting the walk and biscuit that he wants.

Some people learn very quickly and easily how to affect the behaviour of those they live with. Others are never so skilful. There are the perceptive natures whose minds quiver into sympathy with the feelings of those about them, and there are the obtuse who can never be got to understand

5

exactly what someone else is thinking. There are natural gifts in this as in painting or any other art, but that does not mean to say that even natural gifts cannot be improved by thought and study. Those people who deride a study of psychology and say " Well after all it is only common sense " are claiming for themselves high natural gifts. The claim is only occasionally justified.

The history of education affords the most lamentable spectacle of this failure of common sense. Every cruel and repressive method has in its day been assumed to commend itself to all reasonable men. The innate wickedness of children was a religious dogma for centuries, and a careful consideration of children's conduct under the conditions of their lives seemed amply to justify the belief. It was but common sense to control such wickedness with the rod.

The essential difference between the attitude of psychology, and even enlightened common sense, is that psychology alone looks at the problem from inside and asks first of all what it feels like to the experiencer. In a school, how does the child feel under the experience of being taught ? What does he want ? and how do certain methods strike him ? In a works, what does it feel like if someone shouts down the shop every time he wants something sent up ? It may be easy to shout and quite pleasant to the shouter, but how does the man who is shouted at feel, and what effect has this experience on his work ?

So much for the general bearings of the subject. We must say a few words about the sources of information. At first the psychologist looked inward, studied his own mind, and thought all humanity was as he. This led to great errors, because all men are different, and the philosopher is far from being the normal type. But in spite of these errors a large body of useful information was built up, and no psychologist, even to-day, can go far without consulting his own inner life. We can only interpret the experiences of others by comparing them with our own, and we have first-hand information about *one* mind only.

We are therefore compelled to interpret all that we learn of others by our own experience, and the success of our interpretation will depend on how closely we resemble the being studied. It is easier to understand an adult than a little child, a dog than a cat, a mouse than a humble bee. The savage has a different set of ideas from a civilized man and is correspondingly harder to understand. Often the most disastrous mistakes are made by people who are insufficiently aware of the differences between themselves and others.

A little later the close connection between physiology and psychology was discovered and the sense-organs were made the subject of elaborate experiment. We learnt what sounds we could hear and discriminate, what colours were of equal brightness, how fine our discrimination was for weights and tactile space. This was the " new psychology " in the days of William James, and to it we owe the rise of exact methods in psychology. These methods have been applied to various fields and have given psychology a place in industry, the army, the air-force, and elsewhere. Their latest developments, though on rather different lines, are in " mental testing " for grades of intelligence or for discovering special aptitudes for different vocations.

Another line of research was inaugurated by Professor McDougall when he published his *Social Psychology* in 1908. Here for the first time a coherent scheme of man's instincts was worked out, and full use was made of comparisons with animals and simpler types of society. One line of investigation, that of the instincts, has dominated psychology to the present day, and has yielded wonderful results in the work of Freud and other psycho-analysts, notwithstanding their exaggerated emphasis on certain elements in human nature. The comparative method has led to the study of animals and anthropology from a psychological standpoint, and has shown that though man may be the " Beauty of the world ", he is still only " the Paragon of animals ".

More recently still has come the detailed study of human abnormalty and attempts to direct the impulses, particularly of children, into socially desirable channels. Knowledge has grown with the use of it, and the peculiar characteristics of childhood are becoming ever better understood. The child-guidance clinics are spreading over the country and will soon be a most important part of our educational system. It is to be hoped that as the power of guidance of children increases the numbers of the mal-adjusted adults will decrease, and that in time we may be able to control mental disease that is not definitely physiological in origin.

FOR DISCUSSION

1.—What is the Christian teaching on the subject of the nature of the soul ? How does this teaching deal with such problems as those of insanity ?
2.—Compare a vivid dream with a sense experience. How would you try and decide whether an experience was dream or waking ?
3.—Have you ever felt the external world become unreal ? What have you thought of the experience and what have you done to try and restore reality to your normal surroundings ? Have you any theory as to the *cause* of the experience ?
4.—When you say " I didn't really want to do it, but something seemed to impel me." What EXACTLY do you mean ?

BOOKS

PLATO *Republic*, vi. 507 seq. The Theory of Ideas. Cf. also the chapter on Words and Thought in this book.
PLATO, *Republic*, iv. 436 seq. } The Nature of
ARISTOTLE, *Nicomachean Ethics*, i. 13 } the Soul.
Both these books are difficult, but they will repay study. The *Republic* will be referred to several times. It is one of the best and most interesting books in the world. There are many translations. There is one in the " Everyman " Series.
L. P. JACKS, *All Men are Ghosts* ; see especially the story " Dr. Piecroft Gets Confused."
LEWIS CARROLL, *Alice in Wonderland* and *Through the Looking Glass.*

MODERN PSYCHOLOGY AND EDUCATION

PART I

THE DIRECTION OF MIND

CHAPTER I

MECHANICAL *VERSUS* PURPOSIVE ACTIVITY

" I'd have said to the porpoise, ' Keep back, please. We don't want *you* with us.' . . ."
" They were obliged to have him with them : no wise fish would go anywhere without a porpoise."

MODERN psychology, as was said in the Introduction, is characterized by its acceptance of the theory of the continuity of development from animals to man ; but it is possible to start our investigation at either end of the series. We can start by describing the behaviour of the simplest animals and attempt to assimilate the behaviour of complex animals and of man himself to this level, or we can begin with man and try to show how the principles of action, which we observe in ourselves and in those about us, can be employed to explain the behaviour of animals, which, at first sight, appears to be of a very different order.

As will be seen from this book, both methods are used. The actions of men are studied in such a way as to throw light on those of animals and vice versa ; but it has happened that one of the greatest changes in modern psychological thought has been due to a change in the starting point of the enquiry.

Thus, the lowest types of animals, the protozoa, show very simple forms of behaviour, some of which can be imitated by mechanical devices. It is, therefore, possible to argue that the actions of these creatures are essentially mechanical and are determined by their physiological structure. By mechanical action is meant action which follows automatically as the result of the stimulus. As we can exactly predict the movements of a machine if we know its construction and the power which is supplied to it, so, on a mechanical theory of action, supposing we know the exact nature of the living machine, we should be able to predict exactly what its actions would be in any given circumstances. Such factors as will, wish, desire or emotion would have no effect on the resulting action—even consciousness itself would be an unnecessary addition— and there would be no need to imagine that the living creature possesses intelligence or that mental factors affect its actions at all. Certain actions, even in man, are mechanical. A bright light will cause the pupil of the eye to contract, and a sharp tap just below the knee will make the foot jerk forward.[1] Such actions as these are called reflex, and take place without our willing or determining them, and they are very little under our control. If all our behaviour could be similarly explained, the mechanical theory, based on the study of the lowest animals, would be correct.

It has, moreover, been shown that certain of these reflex actions can, in animals, be modified. The introduction of food into the mouth produces a flow of saliva. If, before a dog is fed, a bell is always rung, it is found that after a time the mere ringing of the bell will produce a flow of saliva, even if no food is given. Such a reaction is called a conditioned reflex, since the original behaviour is

[1] Both these are simple experiments. The latter is regularly done by a doctor during a medical examination to test the condition of certain parts of the nervous system ; the reflex of the pupil can be shown at night by setting the subject with his back to the light and reflecting a beam of light into the eye with a mirror

modified by a condition introduced into the situation. In the same way in man many new objects may excite reflex or semi-reflex activities. A child will cry out if hurt by anyone. On the next appearance of this person it may show signs of fear or even cry, although this time it suffers no harm. It has been imagined that it is possible to build up a whole account of man's behaviour in terms of such conditioned reflexes. We should thus have a psychology which took as little account of mind in discussing the actions of man as it does in discussing the actions of the protozoa.[1]

Most people find it difficult and almost degrading to believe that all their actions are the result of the interaction of circumstances and certain specific physiological structures, and prefer to believe that their actions take place in accordance with their will and desires. We are so conscious of the difference between an action such as the knee-jerk, which we cannot control, and that of deliberately setting ourselves to work for half an hour at a Latin exercise, that it seems absurd to rule out thought and purpose in a consideration of the behaviour of man. We think we know why we do a thing, and we take pleasure in carrying out a purpose we have set ourselves. On the other hand, there is no doubt that at any given moment an action is largely determined by previous experience, especially that of childhood. We can " condition " people to like or dislike certain things. To respond in one way or another to certain ideas. Most of Europe to-day is in the grip of governments who are teaching their population how to respond to certain words or ideas, and there is little doubt that as time goes on this process will be carried farther and farther.[2]

But in spite of this we can say that man is not a machine, and in much that he does is actuated by purpose. If, then, we admit the importance of purpose in men's actions, and try to assimilate the conduct of the animals to that of man, we must carry the conception of purpose right down

---

[1] This type of psychology is called Behaviourism. For an exposition of it cf. Watson, *Psychology from the Standpoint of a Behaviourist.*

[2] Cf. Aldous Huxley's *Brave New World.*

into the animal scale. We have seen that it is possible to regard the actions of the lower animals as mechanical; but, on another interpretation of the facts, it is equally possible to regard these actions as the expressions of simple and primitive purposes.

Certain caterpillars climb up shrubs and eat the young leaves on the higher branches; a little later in their lives they climb lower down and feed on the leaves nearer the stem. It is possible to interpret this behaviour as a mechanical response, due to varying sensitivity to light; it is equally convincing to interpret this behaviour as the result of a purposeful search for food of the most suitable kind.[1] If the creatures have a purpose we raise the problem of how definite their aim needs to be. This will be discussed later.

Behaviour in animals as primitive as the caterpillar is really of little use in a psychological discussion, because the fundamental differences in experience must render language adapted to describe our experience misleading when applied to theirs. However, when we are dealing with the higher animals, such as cats and dogs, who live in association with man, we can more easily give an account of their experience which may be correct. We can observe their behaviour easily, and, as it is simpler than man's, it is often convenient to describe it.

Take, for example, the actions of an intelligent dog. It is possible to decide by observation of them, whether they are better explained by reference to a theory of purposeful activity or to a theory of mechanical action.

A dog is lying peacefully in the sun. He gets up, stretches himself, and walks down the garden path. At a certain point his way is blocked by a gate. He pushes against it with his paw, the gate holds fast. He pokes at the latch with his nose, but cannot lift it. He backs off two or three steps and jumps over. Farther down the path he digs up a half-eaten bone and carries it back with him, jumping the gate on the way without trying to get

---

[1] For this and other examples cf. McDougall's *Outline of Psychology*, Ch. ii. You will find there a discussion of these two types of psychological argument. For a still fuller treatment cf. the same author's *Body and Mind*, esp. Ch. xvii. to end.

it open first, and lies down once more in the sun to gnaw his bone.

If we were asked to explain such a train of activity we should say at once that the dog wanted the bone and set out to get it. In saying this we should be speaking in terms of our own experience. If I get up in the night, take a flash-lamp, go down to the dining-room and hunt in the cupboard till I find a biscuit, I do it because I am hungry and want something to eat. We interpret the dog's action as purposive because we know our own action in a comparable situation to be so.

This action of the dog seems to differ in various ways from action which is strictly mechanical, and we know of no machine which would have acted as the dog did. Professor McDougall has shown that there are five main ways in which the dog's activity differs from that of a machine.

(1) It is spontaneous. If a stone is to move it must be thrown ; if a motor is to work it must be started ; but the activity of the dog is not caused by any external event. His movements may, of course, have been preceded by a feeling of hunger, or perhaps a memory of the bone, but such a feeling of hunger or the memory *need* not have resulted in action as it did. If Tom, the son of the house, had lifted the dog up in his arms, then the dog would have been in the position of an inanimate object, and his action would have been motivated by an external force, and would not have shown this character of spontaneity.

(2) The activity is not strictly commensurate in duration with the cause. Supposing a memory image of the bone passed through the dog's mind it would rapidly be gone, but the activity continued for some time after the passing of the immediate cause. With an inanimate object the result either ceases with the cause, as when you press down and then take your hand off a spring, or the effect continues as long as there is no cause to stop it, e.g., a stone flung on the ice continues in movement till friction brings it to rest. The dog's activity does not belong to either of these two classes. It is not merely absence of obstacles which permits the continuance of the activity, for the dog overcomes the obstacles in his path. Walking down a

path, jumping a gate and digging up a bone are not results mechanically commensurate with a memory of a bone.

(3) The behaviour is varied. The dog's behaviour can vary on different occasions when there is, approximately, the same cause in each case. A feeling of hunger might send him into the kitchen, not out into the garden to dig up a bone. Even on the way to the bone there may be variation of behaviour. He will try several ways to get past the gate and we cannot exactly predict which way he will try first. This is quite different behaviour from that of a motor-car when it runs into a stone wall!

(4) The behaviour improves or becomes more efficient in coping with a situation. When, in our example, the dog comes back again, he jumps the gate at once without first trying to open it. He has learnt that the gate is firmly latched. So in most cases we find that animals' behaviour improves with practice. A machine may run more smoothly with time, but it does not learn new helpful movements or drop old ones which have proved unsatisfactory. If this has to be accomplished man has to make the necessary adjustments.

(5) Lastly, there seems to be a natural end to the cycle of activity. The dog wants his bone, goes to get it, and having got it, settles down to gnaw it peacefully, and perhaps in the end goes to sleep again. There is an aim set from the beginning of the activity, and when the end is attained activity for the time ceases. In the case of a machine there is no such obvious end to the activity.[1]

All these marks of behaviour are intelligible only on the assumption that the animal has a purpose. Action begins, apparently spontaneously, when a purpose is formed, and continues as long as the purpose is unfulfilled, even if obstacles intervene. Every variation of behaviour which is of advantage for securing the end will be followed, and when the purpose is accomplished that particular type of activity will cease.

This purposive character is shown in all types of behaviour, and in animals it is rare to see activity, except

[1] How would you explain such apparently purposive activity as that of a crane picking up iron ingots, putting them into a furnace, taking them out again, and passing them over to the rollers?

the pure playing of kittens or puppies, which has not some obvious aim. When a cat is not hunting, or walking about for exercise, or seeking the companionship of other cats, or looking after her kittens, or washing herself, she is generally just sitting still or sleeping. The same thing is true of other animals and of man, though owing to the more complicated life man leads it is often difficult to say what is the real purpose that lies behind some of his acts. Even the small baby seems to appreciate purpose in activity. Thus when you first begin to play " This little pig went to market "—touching the baby's thumb or big toe—the baby looks surprised or cries ; but when once you have gone through the game, and he begins to see your object, he beams with pleasure, and again and again indicates his desire for a repetition. It is possible that this love of repetition of games and of stories in the exact form in which they have been previously told is due to the increased pleasure the child gets when he comprehends the object of the game or story.

To say that all action is purposive does not necessarily mean that the actor is always conscious of the purpose which motivates the activity. We *may* be very conscious of the purpose ; students working for an examination have the aim of their activity very clearly before them. On the other hand, when we suddenly step out of the way of a motor-car our aim is to preserve ourselves, but that aim is not clearly conscious at the moment. We have to act too quickly to have time for thought. We say we " did it before we had time to think ".

The same is true of an adult. Nothing is more infuriating than to be compelled to perform some apparently purposeless task ; but as soon as the purpose is adequately explained the activity becomes interesting. Children in school will rebel against being taught anything for which they do not see a use. The average small boy regards Latin grammar as useless and uninteresting ; but a child who has set his mind on a scholarship and thinks Latin grammar a step towards it, learns with enthusiasm, rejecting all the supposedly " interesting " variations that the teacher introduces for the benefit of the other members of the form.

If we study purposive actions in animals and young children and compare them with those of adults, we can notice various differences. In the first place, experience, knowledge and the use of language all combine to make our aims more definite as we grow older. Prospero expresses this fact well when reproaching Caliban,

> I pitied thee,
> Took pains to make thee speak, taught thee each hour
> One thing or other : when thou didst not, savage,
> Know thine own meaning . . . I endowed thy purposes
> With words that made them known.[1]

We can often see a child passing from the stage of unconscious purposes to that of fully conscious aims. A baby does not know what it wants ; it is unhappy and howls. A somewhat older child, particularly if it learns to speak late, may know what it wants, more or less, but be unable to explain it. When it has learnt to talk it can express itself, get what it wants and so test and refine its desires. A small child often finds difficulty in saying what its purpose or object is, e.g., a child of three will run round and round a table, apparently just " letting off steam " Here the unavowed purpose *may* be the imitation of a train or a horse, but it is more probably the delight which exercise of the limbs gives. This purpose is, in a way, felt by the child, but he could not put it into words. Even an adult may be helped by learning new words and turns of language. A study of psychology and the new names which are thus learnt often lend definiteness to vague longings, which were previously only half understood, and make plainer motives which before were hidden.

In the second place, as we grow older, we are able to work for ends more remote than those at which we aimed when a child. We do not expect to move a small child to virtue by promising him a reward next week. An adult, however, can work for an aim which is several years distant, and the ambitious man may set up a goal which a lifetime will not enable him to achieve.

---

[1] *Tempest*, Act I., Sc. 2. We shall frequently quote Shakespeare and *Punch* in this book. They afford rich material for the psychologist, as also do Gilbert and Sullivan.

As the aim becomes more distant the steps which lead to it become more and more varied and complicated. A small child fails to copy a finished object if more than a few simple steps are necessary for its completion ; a boy a little older will make a fairly elaborate model with Meccano ; a student will embark on a four-year course of study which involves learning several subjects, making a special arrangement of his way of life, and will carry out a most complicated train of activity in pursuit of the aim he has in view.

In children and animals it is probable that most of their actions are dictated by definite but unanalysed purposes. Many adults, even pursue purposes over long periods and yet never make explicit to themselves what these purposes are. The observer may understand easily enough what is the motive behind the action, but the actor has never consciously formulated it. Such implicit purposes have various disadvantages when compared with the more conscious kind. The chief is that so often they could be better achieved by some other method, if the doer had the full knowledge of what he wanted ; and, secondly, there are certain purposes that lead on to action that would almost certainly be repressed if it was clear to the actor why he acted as he did. It is frequently an humiliating experience to analyse frankly our motives for action, but it is also a very salutary one.

Not only are some purposes unanalysed, many are denied by the actor. When we have been snubbed by a superior we sometimes find ourselves bullying an inferior.[1] But we are not usually prepared to accept this explanation of our act. We usually repudiate it as a suggestion deeply offensive to our moral nature and spiritual dignity. Modern investigations into the causes of mental and physical ill-health have shown more and more clearly how frequently a purpose of which we have never been conscious controls our actions. The child who is denied adequate opportunities of self-assertion at home becomes unmanageable in school. The head-mistress, dimly conscious of her own incompetence, nags at her staff for their lack of reliability or public spirit. As will be shown

[1] Cf. *The Rivals*, Act II, Sc. 1 (latter part).

later, every instinct, representing an aspect of one of the great purposes of life, can issue in acts of whose purpose we may or may not be conscious, and of which, if we were so conscious we might or might not approve.

We will discuss the deeper aspects of this purposive nature of activity and thought in later chapters. Here it is worth while to mention some of the educational practices which find in it their psychological justification.[1]

If purpose is an essential mark of the activity of living beings, it should not be neglected in education. A child works far better if he knows the end to which his activity is leading, and in some lessons—especially practical ones—the mistake is often made of giving instructions before the children realize to what end their activities are to be directed. For example, if the children are to make an envelope by marking out their papers and folding them, they should first be shown a finished envelope, and have explained to them the different processes needed to accomplish the aim of the lesson—the making of an envelope. The instructions then become far more intelligible and valuable. The same thing applies to handwork lessons, practical arithmetic lessons, cutting out lessons, and needlework.

The child's activity should not only be purposeful, it should further, if possible, have the quality of spontaneity. If the children cannot be allowed real freedom of choice, they can, at least, be led so to sympathize with the teacher's aim that they accept it as if it were their own. In many lessons, however, real freedom of choice, within limits, is possible. The superstition that all the compositions of a class need to be on the same subject is dying, and so is the idea that all the children in a class must read from the same reading book. In many schools the time table is so arranged that children may work at subjects of their own choice for a certain part of the day,[2] and in many other directions the value of spontaneity of purpose is realized.

If freedom of choice is not possible, a teacher can often

---

[1] You should try to make these deductions all the way through the book. We have not always drawn them explicitly as we have here.

[2] *e.g.*, the Dalton Plan.

lead the class to accept her aim as if it were their own. If the children are required to write a letter as a form of composition, the children can choose the person to whom they write, and may even actually send the letter when the teacher has looked at it.

When the children have been led to formulate or accept an aim, the most satisfactory results are obtained if the aim be reasonably, but not too remote.

Children cannot think very far ahead, but they need to acquire the power of placing their aims at an ever increasing distance. A distant aim generally involves a variety of activities for its attainment and, therefore, gives an experience in foreseeing and planning activitives which is of great value as training for after life. The preparations for a school play will illustrate this point. The aim is one which the children readily accept as their own, and, moreover, it is fairly remote. The older the children, the more remote the event can be and the longer and more elaborate the preparations. The play can be made to motivate various activities, sewing for costumes, carpentering for the stage, electrical work for the lighting, the learning by heart of much matter, singing, clear speech, dancing, a good carriage, and even, in some cases, considerable historical research. If the play is the children's own composition, it involves other things as well, and the final preparation of programmes and the duties of stewards have further educational bearings. It would be difficult or impossible to teach without such a stimulus much that is learnt easily with it.

It is most effective of all if the child can be brought to accept the teacher's real aim in full. A child will not infrequently apprehend that he is being " educated " and regard this education as a desirable thing. The teacher also desires this rather vague aim and pursues it as best he may. If a child can be got to accept it too he will lend himself to the teacher's efforts, even when the learning has no immediate purpose so far as either teacher or child can see. When John, aged 8, is faced with Latin grammar, the teaching serves no comprehensible purpose that either child or teacher could explain. It is, in fact, an interesting historic survival that has somehow got left over from the fifteenth and sixteenth centuries among the mechanics, mathematics and modern languages of to-day. The teacher teaches it because he is told to, the headmaster prescribes it because he thinks it is " necessary ", and, strangely enough, John learns it because it is in some way part of the mystic process of fitting him for an efficient adult life.

This curious system works well enough with clever children. Learning Latin, or similar material, causes them little discomfort, in fact many positively like it ; they have sufficient power of foresight and imagination to accept the remote end of the activity, and they are ready to accept the suggestions of those about them as to the true way of life. It is very different with the stupid or quite unliterary child. He finds learning painful, and his whole being protests against an infliction he cannot understand. In these cases, and they are by far the largest number, teaching must carry an obvious utility, and must be closely related to practical life.

A child can understand what he must learn in order to be a good carpenter or silversmith. He can realize why he must learn certain types of mathematics or geometry, why he must know some chemistry and metallurgy. While the conception of being an " educated man " is quite beyond him, the ambition to be a good workman is ever before him, and lends vividness to his work. That is why the educational atmosphere of a trade or technical school is so stimulating, and why children will learn there subjects that they would only deride if taught under the intellectualized conditions of a secondary school.

FOR DISCUSSION

1.—Discuss the concept of " Education " and say what effect you hope Education will have on the children you teach.
2.—Discuss the main differences in the type of education given in a trade (or technical) school and in a secondary school.
3.—What are the chief differences between the purposes of children aged 5 and 14 ?
4.—Choose some particular action, or course of action, and discuss how far your conduct was determined by deliberate purpose and how far by the irrational results of previous experience.
5.—Consider the relation between your acknowledged and unacknowledged purposes.

MECHANICAL *V.* PURPOSIVE ACTIVITY

BOOKS

[1] McDougall, *Outline of Psychology,* Ch. ii.

T. Nunn, *Education, its Data and First Principles,* Ch. viii.
These are excellent books and, in conjunction with William James's *Text-book of Psychology* (for students of Education the *Talks to Teachers* might be better), should be used regularly with this book. References will not generally be given to them. They should be looked at as a matter of course at the end of every chapter, and the relevant sections found from the table of contents. Those students who find these books difficult might use Bagley, *The Educative Process,* for a more strictly educational treatment of the subject.

[1] McDougall, *Body and Mind,* Ch. xvii. to end. An elaborate defence of Animism.

Caldwell Cook, *The Play Way.* An account of methods which enlist the children's ready co-operation.

Helen Parkhurst, *The Dalton Plan.* An account of a method of school organization which allows choice in the arrangement of work.

Aldous Huxley, *Brave New World.* A most interesting and informative extravaganza.

---

[1] Suitable for more advanced students.

CHAPTER II

INSTINCTIVE ACTIVITY

" Go to the ant . . ."

In the last chapter it was pointed out that the actions of animals and man show certain characteristics of purpose which distinguish them from the actions of inanimate things. This purposive character of action is so universal that it may almost be taken as the essential mark of life. There is nothing living that does not appear to develop according to the law of its own species. If conditions were always the same, the mechanical theory might explain this, but experiments on the developing embryo have shown that, even when strange and abnormal circumstances are produced, e.g., when the growing thing is pressed artificially, if it lives at all, the creature still finally develops according to the characteristic form of the species. It is possible more or less, to explain *normal* development in mechanical terms, but no theory of mere mechanism can well be formulated which will explain development under these abnormal conditions. It seems almost necessary to postulate in each living thing a life force which is itself purposive, in the sense that it leads to activity which can be best described, and most easily understood, as leading to the accomplishment of a purpose ; that is, the development of the creature according to the law of its kind. This physical development is one of the greatest marvels of the universe, and the continuance of each living thing is equally miraculous. From the world about it the creature takes those substances it needs, and transforms them into its own substance, keeping always the pattern of itself. The marvel is so universal that we might almost forget it, without the reminder of the poet.

> It's a very odd thing—
> As odd as can be—
> That all that Miss T. eats
> Turns into Miss T.[1]

No less wonderful is the whole regulation of the body in health and disease ; and for the greater part of our lives, sleeping and waking, in heat or cold, this unceasing regulation and adjustment goes on. We are not conscious of it, we do not even understand it, and yet all these physical processes take place with regularity and success. This control of the development and working of our bodies is purposive and to a pattern—it is also without the sphere of our conscious thought.

Our minds also seem to possess a comparable organization of a purposive kind. There are the main purposes and the actions that are organized to achieve them ; the intellectual powers that co-operate in the achievement, and the special facilitation of learning an action that seems the result of heredity and practice. All of these will be discussed in turn. The whole life of any creature or plant can be represented biologically as a twofold effort, to keep itself alive, and to provide for the continuance of the race. Of the two the latter purpose seems the more important, since many plants die as soon as they have flowered and produced their seed. In animals, too, we find the mother willing to die in defence of her cubs, when she could save herself by flight if she abandoned them. In man and the animals these general purposes of self-preservation and the continuance of the race appear to be served by certain innate tendencies which prompt us to act and feel in a certain manner in certain circumstances. If you are suddenly scared, you run, you say " instinctively ". If a mother sees anything threatening her child she snatches the child up, " instinctively ". These inborn tendencies to act and feel are called *instincts*.

These instincts can therefore be roughly divided into groups, those concerned with the individual, those concerned with the continuance of the race, and those which are con-

[1] De la Mare.

nected with the life of society. This division is not entirely satisfactory, since one of the most important instincts, pugnacity, seems to belong equally to two groups, but this classification serves for a first discussion of the facts.

In the first group of instincts, those connected chiefly with the individual, we may put the food-getting instinct, fear, curiosity, and perhaps anger. In the second class, concerned with the continuance of the race, the sex instinct and the parental instinct. Pugnacity so frequently enters into the operation of these instincts that it deserves a place here also. So also do the tendencies to construction and decoration. In the last group (connected with society), it is possible to distinguish the herd instinct, with the special tendencies of sympathy and imitation, and the instincts of self-assertion and submission.

The difficulty of placing pugnacity should warn us that all classifications of instincts are largely artificial, that the real thing is a relation between a subject and an object, and that this relation is generally complicated, e.g. we seldom find the sex instinct separated from the instinct of self-assertion or submission ; curiosity is frequently tinged with fear, and so on. This point will be discussed further in the next chapter but one.

We are also born with other tendencies to action which are sometimes called instincts, but are more usually distinguished from them on the ground that, though the tendency to action is innate, there is no corresponding emotion innately given. A baby has a tendency to learn to walk, and, as soon as its muscles are strong enough, it learns to stand up and walk. In the same way a child readily acquires speech. So in other animals there are certain actions which the young are either born able to perform, or are born with a very strong tendency to acquire. A chick can peck almost as soon as it is hatched ; a duckling can swim when it first enters the water ; young birds readily learn to fly after a short parental education, and would probably fly in any case, even if their parents did not teach them to do so.

There has been endless controversy over the instincts and these innate tendencies. Some writers, following McDougall, describe as instincts only those tendencies to action that are shared by man and the animals, that are accompanied by strong specific emotions and which are capable of becoming exaggerated in such morbid states as insanity. Others would confine instincts to such innately organized and completely unlearned acts as crying in babies or pecking in chicks. Others again would closely equate instinct with reflex action. There is not much profit in such discussions. If we regard the conduct of man as purposive, all these types of conduct can be understood and appreciated in relation to their purposes no matter how they are labelled.

In the past too a distinction was drawn between instinct and intelligence. By instinct animals blindly pursued their good without conscious knowledge of their goal, but man, a rational animal, looking before and after, pursued his ends by reasoned intelligence. It has become abundantly clear that man is not rational. It has also been realized, as we study animals more, that they have foresight and understanding of their acts. There is no definite line separating man from the animals. The difference lies in the degree of adaptability that is shown by the different species. All pursue the same aims, blindly or with foresight, but some use methods that seem completely stereotyped from birth while others are enabled to adapt their behaviour to very small differences in the situation. We can, if we like, call the unvarying response pure instinct and say that the varied is controlled by intelligence.

Thus, in some insects, the working of the instincts and innate powers appears to be definite and to vary very little with different circumstances. The result of this is that, under normal circumstances, the animal's activity appears nicely adjusted to the aim in view, but if artificial variations are introduced for experimental purposes, the animal may appear to be exceedingly stupid. There is a certain solitary wasp which digs a hole in which to lay her eggs ; she then goes away to hunt for a caterpillar, which she first paralyses by stinging it, and then drags to the hole. Next, she puts down her prey and goes into the hole to see if everything is in order, and lastly drags in the caterpillar, lays her eggs against it and seals up the hole. Fabre, in order to test the intelligence of the wasp, once removed the caterpillar a short distance while the wasp was in the hole. When she came out she looked for the caterpillar, and, having found it, brought it up to the hole once more, and again entered. Fabre removed the caterpillar a second time, and the same thing happened. For as long as his patience held, the wasp never omitted her preliminary entrance into the hole, and so never got her caterpillar safely in.[1]

In the higher animals and man, the organization and working of the instincts is different. The instincts are not specially adapted for dealing with specific situations, but rather they determine behaviour in general classes of situations. They are, in consequence, more variable, and are much more capable of being adapted to fit different and particular needs. This power of adapting behaviour so as to meet specific situations more efficiently is generally called intelligence. It is possible to make a rough scale to illustrate the different degrees in which behaviour is controlled by specialized innate tendencies or directed by a consideration of particular circumstances.

The case of the wasp quoted above shows a failure to adapt behaviour to a particular case ; the study of bees shows a nice combination of the general with the particular. When bees are given wax on frames they always draw it out in the same way into similarly shaped cells ; but if one frame is broken and the comb begins to sag, the bees join the broken comb to a sound one by a number of ingenious arches so as to support the weak comb.

An example from the tailor ants will show a combination of instinct and intelligence with a still larger proportion of the latter. The tailor ants weave themselves houses of leaves fastened together by a thread of silk from the mouth of the grubs, which still retain the silk glands which the adults have lost. Some ants draw two leaves together and then other ants, gripping the grubs by the middle, pass them to and fro between the edges of the leaves, which they thus bind together with threads of silk. Some of the nests are very elaborate in construction and are built with little pillars and separate chambers. But

[1] For a sequel to this story cf. Peckham, *Wasps.*

even apart from these elaborate structures, there are infinite variations in the position of the leaves used, and the special circumstances of each nest are allowed for in a way which we should call intelligent in a high degree. There is an account given by Professor McDougall of an experiment on his dog, Mick, which illustrates the extent to which the activity of an instinct may be overlaid by intelligence.[1] A box was made with a lid, and a lever by which the lid could be raised ; other complications were subsequently added. A biscuit was put in the box and Mick had to open the box to get the biscuit. He rapidly learnt to work the lever, to unfasten a catch, and to overcome other impediments.

In this experiment the most important thing to notice for our present purpose is not the intelligence which the dog showed, but the basis of instinct underlying that intelligence. If a stone had been thrown into the box, the probability is that the dog would have taken no notice of it, at least after the first time. It was the appeal to the food-getting instinct that determined the dog's activity.

This point is important when we come to consider human acts, for nearly all conduct is *motivated* by an instinct, no matter how intelligent the conduct may be. Moreover, there is not really any opposition between intelligence and instinct. Intelligence completes and refines the working of the instinct, but the ends served by both are the same.

We must not, however, think that man's conduct is determined purely by instinct or intelligence. If instincts supply the main aims of conduct, the means by which those aims are sought are largely determined by society and the conditions under which we live. The operation of the food-getting instinct is perhaps the best example of this. At different ages and under different circumstances, men have earned their living as farmers or hunters, by brigandage or trade. In the modern world the most diverse occupations are pursued as a means of livelihood ; and some of us—in particular lecturers and teachers— get a living largely by talking. Yet all these different

[1] *Outline of Psychology,* p. 196.

courses of action are motivated by the same instinct, and in many cases if the pressure of individual need were removed—as in the case of being left a fortune—that particular type of activity would come to an end, because the driving motive would have ceased to exist. The food-getting instinct is not the only motive at work in these cases. Self-assertion plays a part in prompting us to assume importance—and perhaps other instincts are operative too —but these could be satisfied in other ways if our living were secure.

The other instincts are similarly affected by the circumstances of society and by the acquisition by each individual of that body of knowledge which Graham Wallas has termed " our social heritage ". This social heritage is by no means confined to man, though it is far richer and more important in him than in the other animals. When wild animals have been brought up in captivity away from their mothers, it is sometimes possible to distinguish certain parts of this heritage. Otter cubs are taught to swim by being carried out into the water on their parents' backs. Then the old otters dive away and the cubs are left to swim. They are taught this when about three months old, and later are carefully instructed in fishing. An otter, which had been captured as a cub and kept in a hutch, was later left free in an enclosure in which was a pond. At first it hated the water and had to be coaxed into it by means of a dead fish placed on the slope leading down to the water. It would not swim till pushed in, and dived only when it was frightened. For three days it went without food though the pond was full of trout.[1]

We therefore conclude that the art of swimming is part of the otter's social heritage, handed on from one generation to another, although if we simply observed the adult animal we might imagine that his swimming was the result of an instinct. In man the difficulty of distinguishing between instinct and social heritage is much greater, because man has so much longer a period in which to learn, and is born with much less specialized instincts than other animals.

[1] Francis Ward, *Animal Life Under Water*, p. 54.

Making all allowances for such acquisitions from society, it is still possible to trace in man the activity of the instincts and to see their construction and the manner in which they are modified. We will take examples from two prominent instincts, flight and pugnacity, or, to name them from the emotions which characterize them, fear and anger.

Suppose an unarmed man meets a bear on a narrow path. He probably turns and runs away in the hope of finding shelter. We can distinguish two parts in this event (a) the situation of meeting the bear ; (b) the action of running away. We can also, from our own experience, infer a third part intervening between (a) and (b)—the feeling of fear. Thus, in the event, there are really three parts, the recognition of a situation, the experience of an emotion, and the action consequent on the first two. In our example it is clear that the recognition of the situation comes first actually and logically. If this man had a gun, or if he had met some animal, not a bear, which he believed to be harmless, or if he were contemplating suicide, i.e., if the situation had been different, he would have recognized it as different, and his emotion and action, would not have been the same. Similarly the experiencing of the emotion is the necessary preliminary to the flight. If the man saw a bear and were not afraid, he might reflect that bears are generally timid animals, and that this one was probably as surprised as he was and would bolt if he shouted at it. But the feeling of fear was so overwhelming that he did not reflect, but obeyed an innate tendency and fled.

These three parts of an instinct have technical names : the perception of a situation is called cognition (from L. *cognosco*) ; the feeling is the affect or emotion ; the action consequent on the other two parts is called conation (from L. *conor*). In man the cognitive and conative aspects of an instinct may be greatly modified without much changing the emotion which accompanies them.

We can illustrate this from the case of anger and pugnacity. The expression of this instinct is normally controlled among civilized men, and yet the emotion remains strong. The stimulus to anger seems to be any situation in which our desires or purposes are thwarted. A little child will show signs of anger by kicking the cupboard door which he wants to open and cannot ; a mother will become angry if the slightest disrespect is offered to her darling baby, even so slight a disrespect as speaking of him as " it ", for she desires to have him praised. If we are wearing our best clothes and desire to continue looking well-dressed and impressive, it is a hard matter to keep our temper if a maladroit waiter makes us ridiculous by spilling gravy down our backs. Thus the liability of a person to anger depends in part on the urgency of his desires. If we want a thing very much and obstacles are put in our way, anger is very likely to result as our efforts to achieve our desires are thwarted.

In primitive man the expression of anger was probably physical violence, as it still is with a child ; but society has decided that personal combat between members of the same group is wasteful, and, in consequence, a legal remedy was gradually provided to take the place of the blood feud.[1] But even to-day, the instinct of anger will break all bounds, and modern law admits " justifiable homicide " in cases where a man's anger is considered " righteous indignation ".[2]

In modern society it is normally not considered suitable to express anger even by words, and a gentleman, though he may resent an insult, is often expected to ignore it. Between nations, however, the direct expression of anger in warfare is still permitted. What a man may not do to his fellow-countrymen he may do to the subject of another State. The history of international arbitration is the modern parallel to the suppression of the blood feud.

Anger, then, if allowed free play, naturally results in physical combat, but, just as we can have anger without any resulting combat, so we can have combat or pugnacity without a very strong precedent feeling of anger.

---

[1] The transitional period was about A.D. 1000 in Iceland and about 1000 B.C. in Greece. The feud still lingers in Corsica and Albania.

[2] This is a recognized legal plea in France, e.g. in the case of Mme. Caillaux, who publicly shot the editor of the *Figaro* which had attacked her husband. She was tried and acquitted.

The love of a fight is strong, even among Englishmen. This natural tendency to fight is best observed in boys from about the ages of 9–12. Their main use for their fellow-boys seems to be to scuffle with them, and two healthy boys of this age can hardly pass each other on the stairs without starting a contest. This same love of a fight frequently motivates the activities of adults, though the activity resulting from it is not physical combat. This is Anthony Trollope on his relations with Rowland Hill, the great P.O. official :

> How I loved, when I was contradicted (in P.O. matters)— as I was very often, and no doubt very properly—to do instantly as I was bid, and then to prove that what I was doing was fatuous, dishonest, expensive and impracticable. And then there were feuds—such delicious feuds ! I was always an anti-Hillite, acknowledging, indeed, the great thing which Sir Rowland Hill had done for the country, but believing him to be entirely unfit to manage men or to manage labour. It was a pleasure to me to differ from him on all occasions—and looking back now, I think that in all such differences I was right.[1]

Such combativeness is not always for the general good.

We can tell from our own experience, and physiology confirms it, that anger is accompanied by a great output of energy which is likely to be wasteful, despite the excuse of the bad-tempered man, which is common in the North of England, " I do twice as much work in my tempers as you do in your whole life."

The task for education and society is to sublimate, not to repress pugnacity. There are a great many things in this world that need to be " fought " : disease, sin, drink, famine and slums. The reformer, in using military language concerning his efforts, expresses the fact that he carries into this work the spirit and energy of combat ; and this energy is of incalculable value to society.[2] If pugnacity cannot be turned into these socially advantage-

---

[1] *Autobiography* (World's Classics), p. 259.
[2] Cf. Salvation Army hymns and others, e.g. *Onward Christian Soldiers.*

ous channels, it can at least be directed in such a way as to be innocuous. The games of English people are largely combative, and such a game as Rugby football contains most of the elements of the primitive fight, so arranged, however, as to be comparatively safe. Again in mountaineering, a sport in which there appears to be no opponent, the mountain itself assumes the character of a " foe " to be " conquered ", and the natural difficulties of the ascent assume in the climber's mind the shapes of devices of the enemy. William James, elaborating this idea, even went so far as to recommend international games as a partial psychological substitute for war.

These modifications introduced by society into the expression of anger, mainly affect the conative side of the instinct. In fear the greatest modifications take place on the cognitive side. The natural excitants of fear seem to be loud noises, strange moving shapes, physical pain. We can often observe these stimuli affecting ourselves in a quite irrational way, and in a manner not to be explained by our experience. It is hard to suppress a thrill of fear as an express train goes roaring and glaring through a station, even though we know quite well that we are safe out of the way on the platform. In the same way one may be genuinely terrified for a moment by a strangely moving shadow thrown on a wall by a vehicle passing a street lamp. In many cases of slight pain it is the feeling of fear that makes the whole experience unpleasant, for if one reflects on such an experience as, for example, cutting a finger, it is fairly clear that the experience is only *faintly* unpleasant if the element of fear be removed. From this follows the difference in experience between a pain such as that of a not too severe burn which we understand and are not nervous about, and an attack of earache, when we are afraid of the results which may follow. Experience and teaching add many stimuli to these primitive excitants of fear. Young animals are not afraid of man till their mothers teach them to be. Once, when staying in the country, one of the writers found a baby wild rabbit, old enough to walk about, but too young to have learnt the fear of man. He was as tame as a kitten, would let her stroke him, and sat on the table, cuddling up to the hot water jug for warmth. The same fearlessness can sometimes be seen in fawns and other young animals.

The objects which make man afraid are greatly changed by civilization and the growth of knowledge, but our emotions do not always strictly follow our training. We "jump" at a sudden noise, but it is not normal to feel a true sensation of fear if offered water which we suspect to contain typhoid germs, even though we abstain from drinking it. On the other hand it is easy to frighten children with stories, and this is still done by some unwise persons, though less commonly than formerly. The doctrine of hell-fire,[1] which made miserable many children of a generation or two ago, is now seldom taught in its pristine horror. It is unusual now for parents to threaten children with a bogy man or even the policeman, and the use of corporal punishment in schools is decreasing.

The effect of fear may be either flight or immobility. The start which we give at a sudden noise is probably the relic of the reaction of flight, the breathless immobility with which we lie in bed when wakened suddenly from a terrifying dream is probably an example of the other reaction. The effect of fear on a course of action is normally to bring about a cessation of that behaviour. We have often heard and read the avowal: "I thought I heard or saw something, and I was afraid to go on."

It is for this last effect that fear has been, and is, used as a method of discipline. The earliest codes of morals are—like the ten commandments—mainly negative, and they are generally enforced by an appeal to fear ; a positive command generally needs some other incentive to bring about obedience to it.

This state of things is reflected in our own legal system. The appeal to fear is made when men are required to abstain from acts harmful to society, and the strongest appeal, the threat of extreme physical pain from flogging, is reserved for offenders of presumably so brutal a kind that no more advanced motive could be expected to influ-

[1] V. Dr. Isaac Watts, *Hymns and Moral Poems for the Young*, and *The History of the Fairchild Family*, by Mrs. Sherwood.

ence them.[1] But in some men the feeling of fear rouses a keen determination to oppose it. They scorn to live "cowards in their own esteem," and, like Macbeth, will pursue a course of evil rather than feel they have been deterred by mere fear of the consequences. This "daredevil" spirit is seen in schoolchildren. The history of corporal punishment in the British army and navy illustrates the way in which the appeal to crude fear has been abandoned, largely because it was unable to produce the more positive virtues, and also because it proved ineffective as a deterrent, especially with the best men. These men accepted it as a challenge and responded accordingly.

FOR DISCUSSION

1.—Supposing that in primitive man the instincts were a good guide to action, suggest why they are such a bad guide to-day.
2.—Which instincts does society most rigidly control ? and why ?
3.—What part should fear play in education ? and what in the management of the state ?
4.—It used to be said that persecution could never kill a belief. Is that true to-day ? In what ways have modern persecutors improved on the methods of their predecessors ?
5.—If you were the Dictator of Europe what steps would you take to ensure international peace ?

BOOKS

McDougall, *Social Psychology*. This book is most important for the next seven chapters and should be read by all.

Graham Wallas, *Our Social Heritage ;*
        The Great Society ;
        Human Nature in Politics.
    These books give a psychology from the standpoint of a politician and sociologist. They are extremely interesting and should be referred to for many of the succeeding chapters.

Bovet, *The Fighting Instinct.* A study of one instinct and its effect in various departments of life.

Thomas Hardy, *Jude the Obscure.* This novel illustrates the working of many of the instincts.

Saga of Burnt Njal. Shows the state of things in Iceland when the blood feud was giving place to law.

Trelawny, *Adventures of a Younger Son.*

Fielding, *Tom Jones.*
    The beginning of both of these books shows the effect of stern discipline on a fearless child.

A. F. Shand, *Foundations of Character.*

---

[1] Consider the proposed punishment of blackmailers by flogging.

CHAPTER III

HERD INSTINCT

" All we like sheep . . ."

ONE of the instincts which have most influence on the behaviour of man is the gregarious instinct. This instinct is not possessed by all animals, and in man, though all men possess it to a certain degree, it varies greatly in strength. The instinct is, moreover, important because of the large number of subsidiary tendencies which are connected with it. The change from a solitary to a gregarious life must have brought with it not only many advantages but also many new adjustments, and still has a great effect on our lives.

If we look at animals that have adopted a gregarious way of life we can see certain characteristics which distinguish their behaviour from that of those which still pursue a solitary existence, as, for example, a fox or a cat. These characteristics vary according to the ends served by the animal's gregariousness. Some animals form herds for defence, and for that purpose only, e.g., herds of cattle, antelopes, sheep and such peaceful graminivorous animals. Being a member of a herd gives them advantages, that is, they are less liable to surprise, and more able to resist when attacked. One at least in a herd of feeding cattle is sure to have his head raised and to be in a position to detect an approaching enemy. When alarmed, the combined herd, armed with horns and hooves, is well able to repulse an enemy which could easily take a single animal in the rear and kill him. A group of startled Dartmoor cattle, heads down, certainly seem able to repulse any likely enemy ; and a herd of buffaloes can kill an attacking tiger, which would undoubtedly have overcome any single member of the herd.[1]

Gregariousness such as this is the result of fear and does not lead to the type of action which is characterized by what may be called sociability. Galton, in one of his essays, gives a delightful description of this kind of gregariousness among half-wild cattle :

> I am now concerned only with their gregarious instincts, which are conspicuously different from the ordinary social desires. In the latter they are deficient . . . yet the ox cannot endure even a momentary severance from the herd. If he be separated from it by stratagem or force, he exhibits every sign of mental agony ; he strives with all his might to get back again, and when he succeeds, he plunges into its middle to bathe his whole body with the comfort of closest companionship. A herd of these animals is always on the alert ; at almost every moment some eyes, ears and noses will command all approaches, and the start or cry of alarm of a single beast is a signal to all his companions.[2]

This account shows that, with these cattle, gregariousness, though extremely strong, involved little except a craving for the physical presence of the herd, and a certain sensitiveness to signals of warning ; and this is characteristic of herds organized mainly for defence.

Among hunting animals a different type of gregariousness develops. Here the pack is intended for offence, and must therefore possess more effective means of intercommunication and a more highly developed organization for leadership.

In the defensive herd there are very few animals able or willing to take the lead ; in the hunting pack any animal who finds the track of game must give the hunting cry and start off in pursuit, leading the pack. As in the case of the herd, the pack must be sensitive to signals made by individual members, but these may well be of a more complicated kind, to correspond with the greater variety of actions involved in hunting.

[1] Cf. the slaying of Shere Khan in the *Jungle Book*.
[2] Galton in *Enquiries into Human Faculty*. Essay on the " Gregarious or Slavish Instincts ".

In both these types of gregariousness there appears to be little pleasure in the companionship of others. The isolated animal is unhappy, but when joined to the herd he does not appear to enjoy the society of his fellows, nor to associate with them for any other purpose than mere self-preservation or food-getting.

In man also this simple gregariousness occurs. We need the companionship of our fellow-men. This need for companionship may not be accompanied by true sociability, but solitude is insupportable after a certain time. The bad effects of long periods of solitude are well known, and in such callings as that of a lighthouse-keeper special provision is made to counteract them, and a man, after service on a lonely light, is regularly transferred to one where he will be able to have more society. It is also gradually being realized that the disinclination of many girls to enter domestic service is largely due to the comparatively lonely life that a single servant leads. On this same fact depends the severity, as a punishment, of solitary confinement. This is, with the exception of the " third degree," the most definite form of torture officially tolerated by Western civilization ; and its employment during the war on prisoners who attempted to escape emphasized this aspect of it.

In a third type of association, elements that are truly social occur. Monkeys seem really to derive pleasure from each other's society, chattering together and catching fleas with obvious enjoyment. Bees and ants co-operate in so intimate a way in all departments of life, and have developed such a wonderful division of labour, that it seems necessary to believe that their association is really developed to enable them to achieve a fuller life than is necessary for self-preservation or food-getting. Their societies depend less at each moment on a leader because each member has certain specialized tasks to fulfil, and the prosperity of the society depends rather on efficient organization and good individual work than on the intelligence or courage of the leader. At the same time, these societies have much in common with the pack or herd. Emotion spreads through the hive in the same way as through a pack, and there is also elaborate recognition between members of the same society, and a rejection of those individuals which belong to another society. This characteristic is clearly shown by bees ; two swarms will not, in the ordinary way, mix, and a hive rejects newcomers—as every bee-keeper knows.

From these instances it is clear that gregarious life has certain advantages. Living together may aid in defence or offence, or enable the animals to achieve a fuller and more varied life than they could have achieved alone. It also allows the animals who thus live together to develop certain specialized functions while losing others. A solitary animal must be comparatively self-sufficient, while a member of a hive can specialize in one of several ways and have his deficiencies supplemented by others. Thus the worker-bees tend the queen and feed the young, while the queen lays the eggs for the hive.

Gregariousness in man serves all these purposes. He may have developed it to increase his powers of defence against other animals, and later as an aid to his hunting. In any case, to-day the social aspect is the most important, since the whole structure of our civilization is built on the division of labour, and presupposes the assistance rendered by each man to others ; but we can see in the forms of association which exist to-day, marks of all the different types of more primitive gregariousness, and the behaviour of men in different circumstances shows the instinctive tendencies which lie behind their actions.

A simple gregariousness, not very dissimilar to that of Galton's oxen, motivates the desire which many people feel to form a crowd. In most towns there is a street in which the populace walks up and down on Saturday evenings. This activity is much more than a congregating of boys and girls, youths and maidens. Groups of men lounge at corners and chat, groups of women stand about shop entrances, or youths walk apparently idly up and down enjoying the sense of forming a part of the " life " they feel around them. To a spectator it seems the poorest amusement, but apparently the comfort of the experience of jostling crowds of fellow human beings is sufficient to compensate the walkers for the disadvantage of noise, dust and crowding. Men find comfort in the presence of their fellows, especially when those fellows are enjoying themselves, and they have an additional joy in the *evidences* of their fellow-men. Lights and traffic and human noises, eating houses, shops and theatres make a large city the most attractive of places to many people. The chief element in the comfortable feeling is the sense of safety which the presence of, and evidence of, one's neighbours brings—a survival, no doubt, of a similar feeling in members of flocks. A similar liking, though on a slightly more intellectual plane, for being with a collection of people and sharing in their experience, will keep thousands of reasonably comfort-loving people shivering for hours in an east wind to see a football match, and made the Coronation what it was.

If we wish to be with our neighbours we must conform to their standards, and hence the strength of the desire to " be in the fashion " or " respectable ". Peculiarities isolate, and many a youth would suffer considerable inconvenience rather than do a thing which is " bad form ", or is " not done ".

The tendency to form a " crowd " is on a slightly higher level. A crowd is not just a collection of people, it is a body of people with some common aim, however ill-defined. It may be assembled simply to watch a show, or it may be marching to destroy the Bastille, the emblem of tyranny. Such a crowd needs a leader if it is to act, and, if a leader is wanting, a crowd will be absolutely powerless even though it actually possesses the means to achieve its ends.[1] But if a suitable leader is forthcoming, it is capable of actions both worse and better than those which its individual members would perform. Too many writers, when speaking of crowds, have emphasized only their worst qualities. It is true that a crowd will lynch and plunder when an individual would not, and the disturbances of the last few years have afforded many incidents as terrible as the excesses of the French Revolution. The following from the *New Statesman*, February 19th, 1924, is typical of many, and is only remarkable as being

[1] See the helplessness of the leaderless revolution depicted in Merejkowski, *The 14th of December.*

the action of citizens of a state usually well conducted and highly civilized.

An orgy of revenge and murder has just taken place in the little town of Pirmasens in the Palatinate. The Separatists, abandoned by the French, had hauled down their flag and were preparing to withdraw. But as a last act of tyranny and folly they prohibited the reappearance of the local paper, which had been repressed under their régime, and this put the match to the powder-magazine. They found themselves besieged in the government buildings by an infuriated crowd, on whom they presently opened fire. At the end of a few hours the stronghold was burnt out, and the defenders either perished in the flames, or were kicked to death, or beaten, or hacked with sticks and axes.

Against actions such as these we must set occasions when a crowd or a nation is stirred by a wave of self-sacrifice, and in the strength of its corporate feeling performs actions that individuals would have hesitated over for a long time if they had considered them individually. There are many instances of this from the French Revolution and elsewhere, but the nearest to our own experience is the wave of patriotic fever which led so many men to enlist in the first few days of the Great War. Though this was not an action by a crowd physically co-present, the feeling was the same, since the modern newspaper creates its own crowd wherever it is read, even at the most individualistic breakfast-table. This greater violence of crowd action, either for good or for bad, is partly due to the sense of power which the crowd gives to each individual, and partly to the removal of certain habitual checks on individual action, which is due to the sense of being at one with the crowd. This latter point will be discussed later.

When a body of people with a common aim becomes organized it ceases to be a crowd and becomes what may be called a " society ". The word is used here primarily in the sense which it bears in such titles as the " Royal Geographical Society ", and will be extended to cover such bodies of men as the state, army, church, and trade unions. The essential mark of a society in this sense is the possession of an aim and an organization within the group;

without such an organization we only have a crowd, and without an aim there is no psychological unit at all. The possession of an organization enables societies to rise above the level of individuals both in power and in knowledge. A comparatively simple case is that of a trade union or the N.U.T., which, through its numbers, and by the agency of its permanent officials, can make its corporate will felt by the whole nation. Here the power lies in the society as a whole and consists in the ability to cut off indispensable services from the nation ; the *knowledge* residing in the Society is possessed by special members and not by the members as a whole, and its most valuable elements, in our example, are experiences of the correct mode of collective bargaining and of the proper persons to whom to prefer complaints.

A more complicated form of society is the army. In it a very large number of men are arranged in a most elaborate hierarchy. No man *directly* commands more than six or seven others ; but by a series of steps each man is indirectly controlled by all the ranks above him. Besides the actual fighting units, large numbers of technicians are attached to the army, which thus has at its disposal experts in practically every relevant subject. In consequence, as a whole, the army can command not only the physical force of many men and guns, but also technical knowledge such as no one man could ever be master of.

In these days very few men are masters of more than one branch of knowledge—generally they are only expert in some one sub-division of one subject. A man is an "electrical engineer" rather than an "engineer", and, as a result, in any big undertaking, co-operation between experts is essential. For this co-operation an organized society provides facilities. An important consequence of this is that man's activities reach a higher level of efficiency than would be possible if each man acted as an individual and had to practise for himself all the operations necessary for life. Such group work is not, however, always easy, and it should obviously be part of the duty of a school to fit children for co-operative as well as individual effort. The matter will be discussed later in the chapter on thought.

We have said that both societies and crowds have aims, and these aims correspond to different needs in man's nature. Temporary impulses lead to temporary associations ; the more permanent needs give rise to societies with comparatively stable aims. For example, the nation is a society which exists partly to safeguard the individual against internal and external enemies ; the trade union aims at preserving or raising the standard of life of its members ; the church provides religious satisfaction ; a tennis club physical exercise and social intercourse, and so on. Just as a man has many needs so he can be a member of many societies, and in the ordinary course of things membership of many societies causes no difficulty. If, however, as sometimes happens, the demands of two societies conflict, a man will choose to remain loyal to that society which satisfies his deeper need. At the outbreak of the Great War many men were faced by the conflict between their duties as members of a State and as members of an international working-class movement whose aim was avowedly pacifist. In almost all cases the State was preferred, because the danger seemed to threaten existence itself, and this is what the State in the last resource is organized to defend. A man's " choice " may also be due to the greater size and power of one of the competing societies. Thus the nation with its patriotic fervour makes a stronger appeal than the I.L.P., and the social consequences of being a " coward " or being " unpatriotic " are more unpleasant than being false to I.L.P. principles, because the nation is stronger and more able to enforce its will on those who disagree with it. Similar conflicts may arise between a religious body and a social club, or even between two athletic clubs to both of which a man belongs. The same principle holds in these cases—a man will continue a member of whichever body seems to him to satisfy the more important need in his nature, even if that need is satisfied in some other way than by the official activities of the society. For example, a man may join a club rather for the company he meets there than for the tennis, which is the avowed object of the club. For this reason many bodies, among them the church, try to appeal to as many interests as possible. Hence, also, the reasons for organizing social and athletic clubs in connection with the church or school rather than apart from them. Membership of the church or school thus carries with it satisfactions of other needs besides the religious or academic one, and the competition between the many societies becomes less keen.

We can now go on to observe the characteristic behaviour of a society under different circumstances.

First, any threat to the whole body makes the consciousness of the unity of the society very strong. Politicians have long known that a threat from outside is the best means of cementing internal unity, and wars have not infrequently been instigated with this end in view, as, for example, by Bismarck. The same holds true in other cases. It is mainly by conflict with other groups that a group becomes actively conscious of its unity, and its members actively benevolent to each other. The members of an exploring expedition faced with great danger will display a loyalty and self-sacrifice which is far beyond that expected from or shown by men in safer circumstances ; and no athletic club is likely to flourish which does not frequently play matches against other teams. On the other hand to say that we need our neighbours, and that we act with and for them, does not necessarily mean that we love them. If people are forced to live in too intimate contact the usual result is friction. We generally quarrel with our colleagues—especially at the end of term—and are usually glad to see the last of them for three weeks. Group feeling, therefore, is intermittent, and is most satisfactory when the members of the group are separated from it fairly frequently.

A second characteristic of the conduct of a group is the need which members of a group feel to recognize each other. Such recognition will increase the feeling of group solidarity and give pleasure. In consequence of this, a large number of types of recognition are used by different groups. The national groups are distinguished by their speech, and the hearing of one's own language in a foreign country will often cause a strange sense of pleasure and relief.[1]

[1] V. Mowbray's complaint when he is banished ; Shakespeare's *Richard II.*

Within the nation different districts have their own dialects, and different classes their own peculiarities of diction. A very young man about town takes great pride in using the latest jargon of the smartest set. To use certain phrases is to show the badge of one's associates. It is generally possible to recognize by his speech a member of one of the older universities, and a fellow member can generally tell from which of the two the speaker comes— each university clinging to and intensifying its own special idiosyncrasies of diction for this very purpose. In consequence of its extensive use as a means of recognition, mode of speech is generally closely attended to when we are seeking to judge a person ; and the social value of good speech is so great that the emphasis laid on speech training in schools is fully justified. Many other things beside speech are used as means of recognition. There are masonic signs, trade union badges, blue ribbons, and the like. Many bodily habits are also used ; no lady, in the past would go out to tea without white kid gloves, and an American hotel cannot conceive a man to be a gentleman if he does not require the use of a private bathroom.

Thirdly, and even more important, comes sensitivity to the voice of the herd. This in animals is the mechanism by which signs of fear, or desire to hunt are acted upon by all the herd together.

In man three tendencies are distinguishable through which an individual becomes sensitive and responsive to the voice of the herd. These are sympathy, imitation and suggestion, which refer respectively to the assimilation of the feelings, actions and thoughts of the individual to those of the group to which he belongs, and to those of the people with whom he associates.

(a) *Sympathy.*—In a group of men there is often a crude spread of emotion similar to that shown by animals when a whole herd of cattle stampedes at some object of fear. Such a spread of emotion occurs when a panic spreads through the audience in a theatre at the cry of fire, or when a crowd becomes angry and ready to fight, although very few people know clearly what is the cause of the distur-

[1] The whole question is well discussed dramatically in Shaw's *Pygmalion*.

bance. It is not necessary for each member of the crowd to be conscious of the cause of the emotion before he experiences the emotion. The expression of the emotion by those about him is enough to rouse that emotion in him directly, and, in consequence, a panic once started may spread, though there is no real danger. In the same way any injudicious action on the part of the police regulating a crowd may drive the whole crowd to fury, even though only one or two people were affected in the first instance, and few know the original cause of the outbreak. Everyone who has been present at a fervent revivalist meeting has felt the sway of crowd religious feeling ; actors know well when the " house " has become sympathetic and laughs or thrills as one man ; and a good teacher can feel when he has " gripped " the class. Sympathy not only operates in crowds, but also between individuals. A very young child may feel it. A little baby will respond to a smile from another person, but may wail if it hears another child crying ; a gay group of people will raise our spirits, and one obviously tired person depresses a whole party.

For a group to share fully the same emotion certain conditions are necessary. The emotion must be expressed, and expressed in such a way as to be vividly seen or otherwise apprehended by others. This is why emotion spreads best in crowds. If the people are not present together, the spread of emotion depends on the ease of communication or the existence of such means as newspapers for spreading the expressions of feeling.[1]

Secondly, it is necessary for us to feel that the folk with whom we sympathize belong to one—our—group. That group may be transitory, i.e., all classes of people may feel themselves one in the fervent religious atmosphere of a church service. As long as we feel ourselves apart from the group and until the one dominant aim of

[1] Many people who " listen-in " to plays, music, or humorous items do not enjoy the performance as well as if they formed part of an audience in a hall or theatre. This is largely due to the absence of crowd feeling—that delicious sense of being " one " with our fellows. Actors and performers also complain that they cannot do as well when they have not the feeling of response to help them.

the moment has " got " us, and made us one with the group, we do not sympathize with it to the full.

Like charity, sympathy begins at home, and we only gradually learn to extend our sympathies as we realize that we belong to larger groups. For ages the same sympathy that was given to men was not given to animals ; for hundreds of years the slave was outside the range of sympathy of the free man. Many people cannot find it in their hearts to pity the sufferings of famine victims in Russia though they contribute to funds to provide Christmas trees for slum children, i.e., they cannot feel themselves of the same group as the Russian victims. Galsworthy's play *Loyalties* is an elaborate study of the way in which class and social prejudices confine the individual's sympathies to the members of his own group. Nothing does more to widen our sympathies than contact with people of different classes and different countries, because only thus do we realize the common humanity of our fellow-men, and on that basis build up a conception of a world-wide group to which we all belong as human beings. Differences of race or status begin then to seem so comparatively unimportant that we enlarge our group to include them rather than ensconce ourselves within our own particular pale.

Even within the group, however, there is not indiscriminate sympathy. We do not generally catch an emotion unless someone intends to spread it ; a cry of fear or warning will arouse fear in us, or a shout of anger make us join in the fray ; but it is quite possible to stand and watch a fight unmoved, save, perhaps, by disgust ; and gaiety in which we are not invited to share, has a depressing effect.

Similarly sympathy is generally accompanied, in adults, by an intellectual conviction that the object of our sympathy deserves it. Suffering which we feel to be entirely the sufferer's own fault moves us more to annoyance than to pity.

(*b*) *Imitation.*—Similarity of feeling tends to produce similarity of action, so that primitive imitation is closely connected with primitive sympathy. But imitation may happen when there is little emotion present. A baby

46

learning to talk will put his lips in the position in which an older person places his, and, if a note is sung, the baby will sing back more or less in tune. Later the child learns to speak with much the same intonation as its parents, and will catch many tricks of manner from the people with whom it associates. This type of imitation is very largely unconscious and is determined, to a great extent, by the amount of intercourse between the imitator and his model.

There is also conscious imitation. This may be of two forms, differentiated by the aim of the imitator. He may imitate so as to secure the same end as his model, or so as to be like the person imitated. In the first case there is no need for the imitator to have any particular feelings for the model. We may wish to get over a fence, see someone come along, go to a particular spot and, pushing up a bar, crawl through in a particular way. When he is gone we do the same. Much of the imitation used in learning is of this type ; but it is necessary for success that the end should be desired and the steps to that end attended to. Frequently in schools, when we ask children to attend and imitate, they do not desire to achieve the end we suggest to them. Too often under older systems of education the end was actually repulsive ; it is occasionally so to-day, as when the secondary school teacher unwittingly holds herself up to girls in their teens as the type of educated woman which they should aspire to be. In such a case, the disinclination to achieve the end proposed makes the pupils adopt a course of action as different as possible from that which is urged upon them. But, when the end is desired, this learning by imitation is of great importance. It is, indeed, the regular way of learning to perform skilled actions of any kind. A detailed description of what is to be done is very hard to follow when compared with an actual demonstration. Therefore, in most skilled trades, the apprentice period is largely occupied in watching and attempting to imitate the work of the older workmen. A similar purpose is supposed to be served by the pupil teacher year for teachers, while the value of the demonstration lessons given in the training college depends on the fact that example is better than precept.

The second type of imitation is due to a desire to be like the person imitated. This desire may be due to admiration for the power or social position of the model, or to love, which seeks to bring about unity between the lover and beloved. Fashions illustrate the imitation due to admiration. Fashions spread from above downwards. It is the leaders of society who first adopt them, and they are imitated by those lesser in rank and wealth. As soon as the fashions have spread a certain distance the leaders of fashion, not wishing to be like their inferiors, change their style of dressing, and a new period of imitation commences. This imitation is thus completed by opposition, and where one seeks to rise by imitating his superior, the other avoids falling by acting in opposition to his inferior. Fashions in words provide good examples of such changes. Many words, which were once used by the upper classes, have now sunk to the lower.

As *Punch* remarks :

> No one mentioned in *Debrett*
> Talks about a serviette ;

and though in the past a great educational institution might call itself a " Ladies' College ", it would not care to do so now if it were taking a new name. " Lady " has descended in the social scale, and we talk about " char-ladies ", but call our friends " women ".

Imitation based on love has not this double tendency. If we really love a person we generally try wittingly, or unwittingly, to be as like the beloved as possible. We long to share their experiences and their thoughts, to read the same books, to adopt their attitudes towards life. We grow to appreciate their tastes or try to make them share ours. Children learn rapidly from teachers they admire, friends acquire habits of thought and speech from each other, and married people, as the years go on, often grow curiously like each other in expression and even in features. It is therefore necessary in schools to present worthy objects for the children to imitate. Stories of great men will often fire a child's imagination and make him try to resemble his hero, but it is well to select the heroes carefully, or, at least, to choose from their doings those which we really wish to have imitated, otherwise there is danger that a false ideal may be formed.

Imitation is of great importance to society. Not only is it a binding force of great power, but it is also the chief means of handing on to the growing generation the acquisitions of the community. By imitation of actions and the acceptance of beliefs, the child and youth enters into his " social heritage ", and is able, when older, to make his own advances.

Imitation is not opposed to originality unless it is carried too far. An original work to be of value must start from imitation, since it is only through the latter that the beginner can reach the point at which originality becomes valuable.

(c) *Suggestion* is the process by which we accept ideas from others without ourselves having adequate grounds for their acceptance. It is, of course, closely connected with sympathy, because if we take fright and run away, it is because we believe that there is something dangerous to be afraid of. But it rapidly develops beyond that; and many of the beliefs which we accept have little emotional support, and are not traceable—except in a very roundabout way—to the influence of sympathy. Suggestion is too often spoken of as if it were something abnormal; on the contrary, it is one of the most usual things in the world. Very few of the beliefs we hold can be said to rest on really adequate grounds. We believe them because we were told them, or because we imbibed them, without adequate enquiry, from a book. The power of suggestion in the printed page is remarkable. We tend to believe that, because a thing is printed, it must be true. *Punch* has had more than one article on this point, of which the best known is perhaps the story of the husband who attempted in vain to discourage his wife from giving him vegetable marrows for dinner,[1] and finally achieved his end by writing an unsigned article which was published

---

[1] *Punch*, November 12, 1924. Cf. advert. for papers, " 20 million people read this every day ! " The printed pamphlets inside patent medicine boxes, telling in confident terms of the remarkable cures already wrought, have often more power to heal than the actual medicine.

in her favourite paper. This article showed the danger of continuous feeding on marrows, and the wife, deeply impressed by the authority of print, at once changed the menu.

The only adequate ground we can have for most of our beliefs is that our authority for them was a reputable one. If we ascertain this before believing, our manner of belief would not be brought under the head of suggestion. If we accept the belief uncritically we do so by mere suggestion, and our belief may be true or false. The truth or falsehood of the belief, however, makes no difference to the psychological process of acceptance.

The origin of suggestibility determines some of its characteristics. We accept suggestions from the group as a whole, e.g., when we take the " tone " of an institution from membership of it (public schools depend much on this method of education by suggestion), or from someone who impresses us as a leader, either by power, position, learning or some other cause. We are far less suggestible to our equals when acting as individuals and hardly suggestible at all to our inferiors.[1]

Furthermore, as the definition indicates, suggestion is a matter of assertion rather than argument. A cry of fear asserts, not argues, the fact that danger is at hand. The speaker who wishes to sway a crowd, as at an election meeting, deals more with assertion and denunciation than close reasoning. A similar method is characteristic of those newspapers which, from the prestige of a million circulation, claim to speak with the voice of the herd. They have learnt the value of a phrase or slogan, and a single number will contain as many as three repetitions of a point with not a single scrap of argument on any occasion. The newspaper history of our recent relations with France, Germany and Russia affords countless examples of this type of suggestion, while Hilaire Belloc's essay *The Tag Provider* [2] gives, in a humorous form, much of the psychology of the slogan.

[1] Perhaps the wife in *Punch's* story was more suggestible to the printed opinion on marrows, because she imagined the writer to be a person more superior to herself than her husband was !
[2] In *On.*

Frequently a belief, originally accepted as a suggestion, gathers round itself a whole mass of confirmatory evidence. This is due to two causes. We tend to notice and remember what fits in with our beliefs, while we are likely to forget that which does not. In the second place we tend actually to perceive what agrees with our wishes and beliefs. This will be discussed further in the chapter on Perception ; it is a real factor in building up evidence in support of already formed beliefs. Two examples will make this clearer. Shortly after the Russian Revolution a number of books appeared, written by people who had been to Russia and studied the state of the country. Those writers with Labour sympathies gave a far better account of the prosperity and order than did those whose politics were directly opposed to the Revolutionary Government. All the writers were probably honest ; they had noticed and remembered different things. For many centuries the belief in witchcraft flourished very strongly in Europe and America. Thousands of persons were tortured and put to horrible deaths because they were accused of practising it. Their judges were usually honest citizens who had nothing to gain by the deaths of their victims, but felt compelled to act as they did because of the evidence put forward. Here is an example :—

" At the assizes held at Bury St. Edmunds for the county of Suffolk, the tenth day of March, in the sixteenth year of the reign of our sovereign Lord King Charles II. . . . Rose Callender and Amy Duny, widows, both of Lowestoft, were severally indicted for bewitching Elizabeth and Ann Durent . . . Elizabeth and Deborah Pacey, and the said Callender and Duny, being arraigned upon the said indictments, pleaded not guilty : and afterwards, upon a long evidence were found guilty and thereupon had judgment to die for the same ".

The following is a fair sample of the evidence offered. A quarrel having arisen between the old women and the parents of Elizabeth and Deborah, the children became grievously afflicted ; " their fits were various, sometimes they would be lame on one side of their bodies, sometimes on the other. . . . Once they were wholly deprived of their speech for eight days together. Upon the recovery of their speech they would cough extremely, and bring up much phlegm, and with the same crooked pins, and one time a twopenny nail with a very broad head, which pins (amount to 40 or more) together with the twopenny nail, were produced in court ".

The judge thought the evidence inadequate and left the matter to the jury who, in less than half an hour, returned and found the accused guilty on every count, and they were therefore hanged.[1] The children immediately recovered.[2]

A large part of the art of the impostor therefore consists in asking people to believe things to which they are already predisposed, since it is very difficult to make people adopt beliefs which are disadvantageous, or contrary to already firmly established opinions. It is hard for the capitalist to be converted to Socialism, or for the clergyman to accept the arguments of the atheist. On the other hand, suggestions congruent with the general trend of thought are readily accepted. Freemasonry is generally regarded with suspicion in Catholic countries. In 1884 Leo XIII. issued an encyclical against it, and in 1885 a man named Leo Taxil published a book in four volumes containing an exposure of the Freemasons. Taxil was an international cheat and impostor who had been in hot water several times already. He accused the masons of being in league with the devil, of practising the most horrid vices, and of working a telephone by the aid of devils.[3] His book was received with rapture, 100,000 copies were sold, and it was translated into four languages. He received a solemn papal benediction and in 1896 was the hero and saint of a great anti-masonic conference at Trent. He invented a lady, Diana Vaughan, who kept him supplied with information. Apparently he grew tired of the joke in the end, for in 1897 he held a large gathering to meet

[1] Sax Rohmer, *Romance of Sorcery*. This book contains much very interesting matter.

[2] A good example of this was provided on a ship at sea in September, 1935, when a rumour started, and was all over the ship in a few hours that England had declared war on Italy. The only communication with the outside world was by wireless. There was nothing in the bulletin to suggest the rumour. But all believed it.

[3] Telephones were not then in use generally.

this Diana, and then declared the whole thing a fraud. The predisposition of his dupes to distrust Freemasonry had been the condition which had made the fraud possible.

For a modern hoax we may compare the adventures of Jones and Hill told in *The Road to Endor*. The rapid growth of Spiritualism after the War, whether Spiritualism is true or not, was due to the desire of so many people to get into touch with their lost ones.

The fact that *leaders* generally give the suggestion, and *followers* accept, renders many people of strongly independent character very adverse to accepting suggestions from others. Sometimes this feeling is so strong that the people are contra-suggestible and always tend to act in a manner contrary to that suggested. This state frequently arises in family relationships. Many sons are contra-suggestible to their fathers, and nearly all boys are so to their elder sisters. The only way to influence such people is to allow them to believe that they have had the idea themselves, and then they are likely to act upon it. A similar thing sometimes happens in education. A pupil may form a low opinion of the capacity of his teacher ; he is then unlikely to learn anything from him.[1] The pupil must be suggestible to the teacher if endless time is not to be wasted on argument and explanation, but if the pupil feels himself the equal of his teacher this attitude is not likely to be adopted. Some people have this independent spirit so strongly that they are practically unteachable. They will never admit another's superiority, and, therefore, cannot learn from them.

These results of the Herd instinct are obvious, and concern the main external actions, but there are other results which are more difficult to observe and analyse. There seems to be something in the nature of a group consciousness ; an understanding by each individual of the wishes, feeling and intentions of the group. When one watches a flock of pigeons on starting flying together, wheeling wings agleam all in a moment, one imagines

---

[1] V. *The Brook Kerith*, by George Moore, which describes the difficulty Joseph of Arimathea found in learning from the teachers he disliked, and the rapidity with which he learnt from his beloved Greek master.

that each bird obeys a common awareness of intention rather than the signal of a leader. Rivers noted something the same among the members of his boat's crew in the South Seas when everybody always seemed to know, without previous observed arrangement what each would do. So too a Quaker chairman can take "the sense of the meeting". Other observers of men and animals have noted the same thing. There is among us the curious spontaneity and succession of children's games : one day everybody is spinning tops and the next they are all skipping, and so far there seems little evidence as to how the change comes about. In actual daily life there are interesting variations among people in sensitiveness to the feeling of the group of which they make part. Some people are very obtuse, others always seem to know what is going on in the minds of others. There are some people who by experience and will are always part of a group. They wish to co-operate for the good of the group, and their sensitiveness to the group conditions enables them to do it to the fullest extent. There are others who by nature expect the group to be their servant, and either do not feel or ignore the common condition. This selfishness is the product of various causes. A child has to be trained to take his place in the group, and to attend to the wishes of those about him. Some people miss the training, and add to natural obtuseness a failure of will. Others are so convinced of the importance of their own individual purposes that they feel they can ignore suggestions coming to them from outside.

There is a tendency for the educated man to try and resist group promptings. The mass activities of man are so frequently worse than his individual actions, the acceptance of propaganda is so much taking the place of thought, that the intellectual feels it his duty to maintain his individual standards, and his responsible thought in the face of attacks of national hysteria. While there is probably much to be said for this attitude, such a man finds himself too often in an uncomfortable position. He is isolated and made the object of persecution. But even the ordinary man is often too much of an individualist for complete comfort. Perhaps if man were a completely socialized insect like a bee, it would all be simple and the " voice of the hive " would carry complete authority. When one is dealing with a beehive it sometimes happens that a bee flies straight out of the hive, alights on the first part of the intruder he can see, and stings him. The result is that the bee perishes. Watching a bee thus sacrificing itself for the public good one can feel little doubt that it has been sent to do this particular work and perish. The writer has often wondered about the thoughts and conditions of this insect hero, and hoped that in such a socialized community the feeling of individual worth and existence was faint. A man in a similar position is normally acutely aware of the conflict between his individual existence and the claims of the community. There are just a few moments of intense excitement when this conflict vanishes, and this is part of the spiritual peace and exultation that some men have found on the field of battle.

FOR DISCUSSION

1.—Study the spread of some belief among a group of people.
2.—Is there any real justification for the opposition between imitation and originality ?
3.—Is it important in a society for there to be "individual thought "? Supposing that the individuals think " wrong ", what steps should be taken to make them think " right " ?
4.—How would you attempt to lead the very selfish child into more social ways of thought.
5.—What can you do to train and direct a child in developing social sympathies ?
6.—How can one foster the spirit of co-operation in a small group ?
7.—What are the dangers and advantages of group competition in schools ?

BOOKS

TROTTER, *Instincts of the Herd in Peace and War*. This book is interesting, if a little uncritical.
LE BON, *The Crowd*. Mainly a study of the crowds of the French Revolution.
[1] McDOUGALL, *The Group Mind*. Discusses the organization of societies as well as simpler groups.
RUDYARD KIPLING, " The Disturber of Traffic ". In *Many Inventions*. A study of the demoralizing effect of loneliness in a lighthouse keeper.

---

[1] For more advanced students.

HUGH WALPOLE, *Mr. Perrin and Mr. Traill.* A novel of school life, showing the way people " get on one another's nerves ".

GALSWORTHY, *The Skin Game.* A play illustrating the way in which social snobbery limits our sympathies.

TARDE, *The Laws of Imitation.* The nature of imitation and suggestion.

DEAN SWIFT, Fable of the Bee and the Spider, in *The Battle of the Books.* A discussion of the part played by imitation in originality.

M. KEATINGE, *Suggestion in Education.* The use the teacher can make of his power of suggestion.

FISKE, *Witchcraft in Salem Village,* one of the most remarkable stories on record.

CHAPTER IV

HERD INSTINCT—LEADERSHIP AND FOLLOWING

" Art thou officer ;
Or art thou base, common and popular ? "

IN connection with the herd instinct, two tendencies exist which are of so much importance that they are frequently spoken of as independent instincts : the tendencies to give and to take a lead, to act as leader or follower. Most men seem to possess both these tendencies, and to display the one or the other on different occasions according to circumstances. In some men one tendency is much stronger than the other, and colours the greater part of that person's life and acts, but it is rare to see one tendency alone manifested in all circumstances. Each tendency is accompanied by a special emotion which may be pleasant if gratified, unpleasant if checked, and may turn to anger if suddenly thwarted.

In a primitive society the leader of the tribe or clan had certain functions, as general in war and judge in peace, which demanded physical and mental qualities of a special kind. Height and strength and good looks, as indications of health and power, were regarded in consequence as kingly qualities. Saul was of ruddy countenance and a head taller than all the children of Israel, and these qualities were part of his qualifications as king. The ruler in peace, e.g., Samuel, was often an old man who had accumulated the wisdom of age and could be relied on to give right judgments.

We still allow prestige to these qualities. We respect those older than ourselves so long as age has not impaired their judgment, and a fine physical presence seldom fails to have an effect. In proportion as we respect size and strength—even though we do it unwittingly—we find it hard to respect at first sight the pasty-faced, squeaky-voiced little man, who may, indeed, easily become an object of ridicule. The joke of *Punch's* drawings of big women with small husbands often lies in the emphasis on the insignificance of the man, which a reversal of the normal size relationship between men and women brings about. We also respect the *signs* of leadership, and fine clothes and other external signs of wealth and power confirm the respect which a fine physique invites, and we may even dispense with the primitive conditions of leadership, so that, when backed by authority, the most unlikely people can become awe-inspiring. Thus the paraphernalia of state officials is a necessary and useful support to their power.[1] The mere suggestion of power will often determine obedience even when real power is lacking. An officer with a confident manner may quell the movements of mutinous troops, though his whole power lies in their obedience.[2] In the same way a very small measure of fear will often influence our conduct to a large degree. The head of the institution to which we belong possesses certain powers over us. We may not be continually conscious of his power to dismiss or promote us, but the fact that he possesses it colours our whole attitude to him, and renders us suggestible and deferential to him in various ways.

Further, to be a successful leader, a man needs to stand in a certain relation to the group which he leads. He must be in sympathy with it, but yet a little in advance of it. He must in some measure anticipate its wishes. A man may be too original to be a good leader. He may see too far into the future and propose measures and hold beliefs which will be accepted in a generation or two, but which seem quite alien to his own time. Shelley was a man of this kind. When he died in 1822 he was practically unknown, or known only to be reviled. When his friend Trelawny died in 1881, Shelley's poems had been

---

[1] Many lecturers feel much better able to face their classes if they are wearing an academic gown.

[2] Cf. various instances in the Indian Mutiny.

reprinted and the advanced literary opinion of the day admired them greatly. By this time many of Shelley's ideas, which were so violently attacked in his own day, are commonplaces of thought. They have been absorbed and become part of the national culture.[1] Tennyson, on the other hand, stepped almost at once to a place as leader of thought in his own generation when, after his ten years' silence, he published his poems of 1842. He had not a new message, but he expressed one which was " in the air ". If to-day we find his thought old-fashioned compared with Shelley's, if we recoil from the Victorian sentiment that permeates it, it is because Shelley possessed a far keener mind than Tennyson, and one which was too noble to be bound by the prejudices of any one age.

The successful leader must not only be in touch with his followers intellectually, he must also be felt to be one with them emotionally. The most successful political candidates are those who appeal to the electors on the basis of common needs and interests ; they seek to emphasize the fact that they are interested in children, play golf like everyone else, would understand local needs, and so on. This has to be accomplished without loss of dignity, and it is only the common characteristics which are accounted creditable that are claimed. No candidate parades his liability to bilious attacks or his dislike of having to work for his living, common though these characteristics may be. The difficulty of the art of leadership consists largely in the necessity of being at once dignified and human.

The position of leader has great attractions. Quite apart from the extrinsic rewards of leadership the leader experiences a certain pleasurable emotion which springs from successful self-assertion. This pleasure of command is one of the attractions of the teaching profession, and it can be tasted very purely in lecturing to a class of attentive students. The misery of trying to instruct an unruly class is also due to the same cause. Here the tendency to self-assertion and leadership is thwarted

---

[1] e.g., his views on the social necessity of the freedom of women, the danger of tyrannous behaviour to children, the evil consequences of bullying and flogging as practised at Eton in the early nineteenth century, and the fact that luxury is not good for trade.

and the pains of a frustrated desire are added to other worries.

Actual leadership is not the only thing which produces the pleasures of gratified self-assertion. Any circumstances which enhance our feelings of self-importance, or which win us the favourable regard of our fellow men have the same effect. A place on a platform at a public meeting will do this for many, and in consequence the giving of platform tickets is one way of conciliating political supporters. Fine clothes are a great assistance to our good opinion of ourselves. There is a story of a Frenchwoman who remarked that " a really well-fitting frock gave a sensation of peace and well-being that religion was powerless to convey ". To a woman, of course, beautiful clothes often mean actual power from an enhanced sex attractiveness.

Occasionally the feelings produced by a public position are so strong as to defeat their object. The amateur about to enter the stage is sometimes overwhelmed by stage fright, and many inexperienced speakers, when rising in a debate, are so excited by being the object of attention that they can hardly say a word.

As in the case of the unsuccessful teacher, a check to the feeling of self-assertion is painful. This check may be due to some accident such as slipping on a piece of orange peel, or it may be due to the hostile or disapproving attitude of our fellow-men. Disapproval is frequently followed by definitely painful consequences and is, therefore, feared, but even without the threat of these consequences, disapproval, in itself, is unpleasant because it acts as a check to our self-esteem and prevents the realization of our desires. The experience of this painful inferiority is part of every normal person's training. From it he learns to respect public opinion and to conform to social codes.[1] The effect is all the stronger in the majority of people because a definite or indefinite fear is added to the painful experience of being disapproved of.

Occasionally an individual seems to escape this social discipline, either through the chances of birth, or an

[1] It is part of every schoolboys' training and of the training of everyone who has social aspirations.

unwise upbringing. A recent case in America illustrated the state of mind of persons who, apparently, had never had to submit to the approval or disapproval of others. Two lads, Loeb and Leopold, the sons of millionaires, and of exceptional brilliance, plotted the murder of a school-fellow. It was intended to be the perfect crime, and was undertaken, apparently, in the search for a new sensation. The murder was duly carried out, but the crime was not perfect and they were arrested and tried. The most interesting feature of the case was the conduct of the boys during trial. They appeared to enjoy the enormous publicity of the affair, and, so far from showing any signs of remorse or even nervousness, daily read all the press reports, gave interviews to journalists, and made themselves shows to an amazed nation.

Very different from enforced and unpleasant submission is the exercise of the genuine instinct to follow,. or take a lead from another. In any herd or pack, if one is to lead, the others must follow, and the one position can be as pleasant as the other ; both are equally necessary and society demands good followers as well as good leaders. There is, indeed, as great an art in being a subordinate as in leading. Most people, of course, stand in both relationships, and are leaders to one set of people and subordinate to another, as a teacher is a leader to her class and a subordinate to her head-master. The good subordinate needs the power to apprehend ideas quickly, the willingness to accept them, and ingenuity in carrying them out in detail. He needs to know when to make suggestions himself and when to refrain. He needs to catch the fire of enthusiasm from another, and to develop principles to fit particular cases. Like every other human relationship this one has difficulties, and these are best surmounted by conscious and deliberate thought about the situation.

As there are some people who are never happy unless they are in a position of command, so there are others who do not wish to hold any other than a subordinate place. These people shrink from the necessity of decision and the weight of responsibility that a leader must face. Such a character is found among men ; it is commoner among women. On the staff of a girls' school curiously few of the assistants *desire* the greater salary, dignity and freedom of a headship. They cloak their unwillingness under the plea that they so love class teaching that they would be loath to relinquish even a part of it. The real reason is that they will not face the responsibility of leading in a school.

The fact that women are more unwilling than men to assume openly a leading position, is probably due to the connection between sex and the instincts of assertion and submission. We have said above that the instincts do not work in isolation. In sexual relations the dominant part is played by the male, and the female resists his advances to be in the end overcome. Thus the tendency to submission is stronger in women, and is often increased by a training in which girls are made to give place to boys, or sisters to their brothers, with the result that many women are not only incapable of leadership, but take a kind of perverted pleasure in self-sacrifice and submission to " duty ". Such a woman sits up late correcting, with meticulous care, exercise books that might just as well be done in class ; she distributes her hours of work in the most uneconomical way, and seems to be satisfied only when she has made herself ill. This particular type of folly is not confined to women, but it is so much commoner among them than it is among men that it has frequently been assumed to be characteristic of the sex.

There is, however, a further complication in this state of mind. If power cannot be achieved directly, it can often be attained indirectly, through a pretended submission. In sexual relations a woman submits, but by so doing she frequently gains a considerable increase of power. In many happy homes the wife really rules through her capacity of flattering the husband and making him accept her views as his own. This desire for power often appears as another type of self-sacrifice, as dangerous as the one mentioned above. The woman begins to fancy herself indispensable. She cannot imagine her children safe or her husband comfortable if she herself does not pour out the tea or bath the baby. In professional women this tendency, denied a more amiable outlet, manifests itself in a fussy exactitude and an overwhelming " sense of duty ". It is impossible for a lecturer to stay in bed for a day with a cold because of the loss to her class if she fails to teach them. The head of an organization cannot attend to family business because there will be no one to sign letters.[1] Both suffer and impair their real efficiency and power, because they pursue a shadow and do not know that they do it.

Children are in a particular position in relation to the instinct of self-assertion. They undoubtedly possess it from a very early age, but they are handicapped in any expression of it among adults by their small powers and their mental immaturity ; in consequence to a strongly self-assertive child childhood may be a period of considerable misery :

> Be gentle to the young, for they've enough to bear.

There are many devices by which a child seeks to assert itself—it may be naughty and break out into violent fits of temper ; it may whine and complain and refuse to eat its food ; it may develop unusually virtuous and studious habits and become a little prig. The way to deal with these types of conduct is mainly to deprive the child of the satisfaction that it hopes, unconsciously, to gain from them. The child who will not eat its meals draws the attention of the whole family to the struggle, and usually gets fed between meals to " keep up its strength ". If the refusal to eat is ignored and the child only fed at proper meal times, the charm of the situation is gone, and, as no child would allow itself to starve in the sight of plenty, it will, after a day or two, start to eat normally once more. In the same way a child who gets no approval for its conceited remarks or affected diligence, loses such habits, and the child with the violent temper can gradually be made to see that politeness will usually accomplish more than fury ; and when once this has been really understood a reformation follows, and the instinctive

---

[1] Cf. E. M. Delafield's very unkind and very clever novel, *The War Workers.*

reaction to opposition, anger, is replaced by one which achieves better the real end proposed.

These types of self-assertion are more characteristic of the slightly abnormal child than of the normal ; fortunately the majority of children adapt themselves fairly well to their position. They are dependent on, and suggestible to, their parents and teachers, and assert themselves in the company of their equals. In addition most children receive opportunities of self-assertion, even among adults. At home they express their opinion, for the doctrine that children should be seen and not heard is largely dead ; they are allowed to busy themselves importantly about small tasks ; and they show off their little accomplishments without reproof. One small boy once walked into a tea-party, and, stumping gravely across the room, remarked, " I can walk, and I can talk." This is the natural pride in achievement, and the pleasures of it are a definite and desirable incentive to further effort.

In school, also, modern methods give many opportunities of self-assertion and display within the limits of the law. Children may be monitors, group leaders, prefects and games captains. They are allowed to recite to the class, to come out and write on the board, to act in little plays, and to do many other things which satisfy their desire for prominence. In consequence there should be no need for the child whose instinct of self-assertion is strong to seek to satisfy it by rebellion. The rebel is most frequently the leader to whom society allows no outlet, and, in consequence, he throws himself into activities which are directed against the repressive society. The following is a singularly frank account of the resistance to authority by one of the famous rebels of the last century.

My brother was tractable, mild, and uncomplaining. I was in continual scrapes. I insisted on following the bent of my inclinations ; and opposition only sharpened my desires . . . I hated all that thwarted me—parsons, pastors, masters. Everything I was directed cautiously to shun, as dangerous or wrong, I sought with avidity, as giving the most pleasure. Had I been treated with affection, or even with the show of it, I believe I should have been tractable, mild and uncomplaining. Punishment and severity were the only marks of paternal love that fell to my share, from my earliest remembrance.[1]

The violence of rebellion is usually greater when there is strength and merit of character behind it. The weak and worthless bear tyranny mildly and uncomplainingly, while the nobler rebel. In consequence society suffers a double loss, it suffers from the attacks of the rebels and is deprived of its ablest members. This should always be borne in mind when dealing with children. It is generally worth while to discover the cause of, and to try and cure persistent naughtiness, because in many cases the naughtiness is the result of some imagined or real injustice which could be remedied by the teacher, and the character from which it springs is often one which, if rightly developed, would be of considerable service to the community.

The most extraordinary example in history of the continual loss to the state of the ablest citizens through repression is to be found in pre-revolution Russia. For several generations all the ablest and most public spirited of the youth were sent into exile for agitation. To be young, and to have the nobility to detest tyranny, and the courage to give expression to this detestation, was a certain prelude to exile or death. Almost all those who made the revolution learnt their business as revolutionaries, and forged their theories in prison or exile. They were bitter men who had been taught to hate. Those who stayed at home and accepted the Government régime lost hope and self-respect. The result is written at large over all the literature of the pre-revolution period, and the history both before the revolution and after shows the dreadful social effect both on the government and on its opponents of this loss of potential leaders.

FOR DISCUSSION

1.—Give an account (similar to the one in the last chapter) of the working of some other instinct, i.e., curiosity. Show the objects which arouse its manifestations, and the part which it plays in society and education.

---

[1] E. J. Trelawny, *Adventures of a Younger Son*, Ch. ii., init.

2.—Study any self-assertive child you know and show what form the self-assertion takes and how it may be satisfied.

3.—Study the career of any revolutionary leader and show how his views developed.

4.—Explain your own ambitions to leadership and show how you think you may achieve them.

5.—Discuss any leader—in politics, thought, religion, etc.—you admire, and say what it is that attracts you to him.

BOOKS

ORDWAY TEED, *Instincts in Industry*. Discusses the instincts as they are exhibited under industrial conditions.

For SHELLEY see MAUROIS *Ariel*. A life of Shelley written like a novel. The early chapters show his life at Eton.

For TENNYSON, HAROLD NICHOLSON, *Tennyson*, a good life of the poet.

ST. JOHN ERVINE, *Mary, Mary, quite contrary.* ⎱
EVELYN WAUGH, *A Handful of Dust.* ⎰
   Studies in selfishness : the first pleasant, the second most unpleasant.

DICKENS, *Oliver Twist.*

For Czarist Russia :
   KROPOTKIN, *In Russian and French Prisons* ⎫
   DOSTOIEFFSKI, *The House of the Dead*   ⎬ The threat.
   LEONIL ANDREIEV, *The Seven that were hanged* ⎭
   TURGENEV, *Rudin*   ⎫
          Virgin Soil   ⎪
          Smoke   ⎬ The Result.
   DOSTOIEFFSKI, *The Possessed*   ⎪
          The Making of a Revolutionary ⎭
   L. TROTSKY, *My Life*, Vol. I.
   J. STEINBECK, *Maria Spiridonova.*

CHAPTER V

THE STATE AND WAR

In peace there's nothing so becomes a man as modest stillness and humility. But when the blast of war blows in our ears. . , .

WE said at the beginning of the chapter on instincts that the division into separate instincts was made for convenience and exposition and that in practice they worked together. We can see vividly the interaction of differing impulses if we consider such an institution as the modern nation state and its activities in war. For us to-day such states are the most important political fact, and the struggle to bring reason to bear both on the state itself, and in the relationships of various states, is the peculiar task of the rising generation. If they can succeed where the elders have failed there is some hope for the future.

It is difficult to know how the state began. The simplest people that live in the world to-day have no state, no government, no law. They are peoples like the Vedas in Ceylon who live by hunting and collecting fruit. They wander about in small family groups, have hardly any clothes, the rudest shelters, and practically no possessions except a few hunting weapons and cooking-pots. If we can believe the observers they are completely virtuous, faithful to their wives, kind to their children, attentive to old age, and absolutely peaceful. Other simple people seem to be almost as virtuous. The suggestion has been made that sin entered with agriculture, with greater concentration of population and the gathering of possessions.[1]

There is no doubt that primitive peoples possess a sense of the group, however small it may be. They can combine for common purposes and they agree amicably on a common life. It is a group spirit, free from competition and con-

---

[1] G. Elliot Smith, *Human History*.

tention, as it might exist in a flock of migrating birds. The quality that has most struck observers is the peacefulness of these people, their lack of the spirit of competition and contention, and their willingness to tolerate strangers. So long as the tribes are few in number this peacefulness remains. Fighting first appears when the pressure of population begins to make the exclusive possession of hunting grounds important. Hunting tribes need a large territory as there must be room for the game ; and if the game begins to grow scarce strangers are violently resented, or there may be attempts made to extend the territory. This territorial occupation seems to exist in animals ; a dog resents a stranger on his land ; and even birds are said to assert, in song, their rights to a given area. Man in the hunting stage may fight for a district, as he may in the pastoral stage, but in both cases he is mobile, his possessions are few, and he may be as willing to shift his quarters as to fight. A very good example of this attitude was given by the Boers in South Africa, and their continual moves north to escape a government that they disliked. They only fought when they could not easily move farther.

Pugnacity therefore enters the state first in defence of the food supply and for the preservation of life. It comes hand in hand with fear, and the association has remained through the ages. But very early it took to itself another companion, property and the glory of possession. The agriculturist is in quite a different position to the hunter or the owner of flocks and herds. He owns the land itself, and he is fixed to it by his house, his crops, his mass of material possessions ; and very rapidly also by sentiment. He owns the land, and the more land he owns the more things he can grow, the more corn he can store, the more children he can feed, the more secure he can feel in times of scarcity. The passionate peasant hunger for the land springs up. The peasant morality based on the ownership of possessions. The life of stationary toil has come into being. To the group spirit is added the idea of territorial possession, and to the idea of the family the sanction and binding force of material possessions. All this pugnacity must defend, and men begin to die for their country.

Somewhere, perhaps in Egypt,[1] a family invented the divinity of kings. The idea of a divine race, sent to earth to rule, spread by degrees over the world. Europe accepted it early, and traces of the family, the children of the Sun, can be found in the Islands of the Pacific or in America. These kings were different from the local chieftains, who were men among men and held sway by wealth, physical prowess, or ability. They were gods on earth, and with them the state had a new sanction. It was the outward dignity of the divine ruler who gave it unity and meaning. We have still not discarded the idea, and speak of the monarchy in England (admittedly incarnate in a mere man) as the true Bond of Empire. Loyalty to a reigning house, an idea that becomes more and more empty the more it is examined, has been powerful enough to send thousands of men to their deaths, to break up families and squander wealth even in so comparatively democratic a country as England. We have had one civil war fought largely on that issue ; we were prudent enough to avoid a second ; but even to-day there are bodies of monarchists in certain European countries who are eager to plunge their countries in ruin in the hope of living once more under the firm rule of their true sovereigns. War thus becomes the ally of yet a third idea.

Under certain monarchies war is the chief occupation of the state. The Zulus under Chaka and Dingaan lived for fighting. They ravaged the lands of their neighbours, stole cattle, and murdered the inhabitants of the villages they captured. The slaughter at home was little less than that abroad. An unsuccessful impi would be condemned to death, and as the warriors marched, rank after rank, over a precipice to their death, their hearts were doubtless filled with a strange mixture of pride and resignation. It seems almost incredible to an outsider that those troops should not have turned in spontaneous mutiny on their murderer. If they did not do so it must have been that they fundamentally sympathized with him, and accepted his point of view as their own.

There are undoubtedly special pleasures of combat, special virtues of a military life. There is, if one may believe

[1] Perry, *Children of the Sun.*

those who have experienced it, a terrible joy in killing, an enlargement of spirit, a great glory. Chaka gave to his warriors this supreme experience. There are also the virtues of fortitude, loyalty, obedience, the reliability of the disciplined man, the high spirit that has passed beyond the fear of death. The impis that marched to their doom were obeying the law that they had learned and accepted as part of their glory as warriors.

War and the accompaniments of war thus play a great part in the development of cohesion and order in a state; and in fact war and religion are in many cases the real forces for culture. Religion gives the impetus to art, war to all the useful arts. Metal work, road making, maps, engineering, all have their impetus in war rather than in peace. Physical culture becomes supremely necessary in a fighting race; even music has its place in the military no less than the religious life. Even in our modern civilization, war proves the most valuable stimulus to progress. We owe such diverse things as women's suffrage and the *Queen Mary* to the excitement of war or the threat of future attack. The production of oil from coal, the proper drainage of the fen lands, the establishment of adequate playing fields for the nation, all are urged as military measures of immediate or remote usefulness. The war between Bolivia and Paraguay turned a virgin swamp into a country with roads, motor transport and air services. The terrible stimulus of war breaks down long-established habits of conservatism, forces men to face problems anew and is a continual challenge to their ingenuity. Those men who speak as if every soldier were a "man of blood" or mentally deficient have not really understood the position.

It is the special task of this generation to try and find some end to international war. It is no good representing war as something contemptible and wholly bad. It is an activity that has all these merits and causes, and the causes being complex it can have no simple remedy.

War being thus the product of a very complex group of causes can have no simple remedy. It is not enough to say that war is due to a "pugnacious instinct" and that this pugnacity can be sublimated into harmless channels by football and international games. War has become part of the ideas of modern nations and certain situations regularly call this idea into action. But there is no doubt that this idea can be got rid of, at least between certain peoples. The U.S.A. and England have been at war in the past, but of recent years the idea that they might ever be again has faded from our minds. Neither party has the smallest intention of using war as a part of national policy. They can imagine no situation arising that would not be dealt with by peaceful negotiation. A similar state of mind exists among the Scandinavian races. They have disputes, and refer them to the court at The Hague. England and Ireland have recently entered on a new phase. They have decided not to fight each other, and, though their feelings are heated, they content themselves with taxing each other's exports.

A cynic has observed that it is easier to feel pacific towards a country when you know he would beat you in a war. That might account for our harmony with the U.S.A., but not for our forbearance towards Ireland. Nor is it even generally true. A rival nearly equal in power and pretentions may be attacked, while an insignificant state is protected.

The real fact, however, is that modern war is an affair of the politicians. It has passed completely beyond the realm of any type of natural action. A deliberate personal threat or affront produces anger and, possibly, some kind of retaliatory action. The threats and insults of an international kind are so remote, so much a matter of diplomatic routine and precedence, that the ordinary man knows and cares nothing about them till a newspaper campaign, government inspired, tells him that he is furiously angry and in immediate danger. Then he goes about thinking how he would love to " Hang the Kaiser " or perform some personal act of vengeance. Instead he is caught up and made part of a machine in which all personal enterprise is extinguished and he comes to regard his immediate " enemy " as a poor devil as helpless as himself.

We do not need substitutes for war as if war were a natural and necessary part of our lives. We need to acquire a different outlook, one that regards it as simply impossible, a madness that has passed from us as completely as the public burning of witches. If the ordinary inhabitants of a country were left alone that would soon happen. It is the politicians with their ideas of national honour, greatness, and in some cases a half-insane imagination of glory that will not let this idea die.

Part of the politician's excuse is that in the past it has been so difficult to bring about any important change without war. Until recent years there has been no international body that could assist in the settlement of disputes or help a growing nation to find some means of expansion. Such episodes as the settlement of the dispute over the Sanjak of Alexandretta are enormously facilitated by the existence of a common meeting place and a body of impartial opinion to act as intermediaries. At present this organization tends to be successful only in those cases where very violent feelings have not been aroused. There must be a willingness to compromise, an aversion to making war a normal instrument of policy. Where this state of mind exists there is every hope of peace. Where it does not there is little.

Part of the power of governments lies in the suggestibility of their peoples. A nation believes what it is told if it is told sufficiently often and clearly, and there seems little doubt that we are growing more easily influenced by propaganda. This may be due to our education or it may be due to a greater skill on the part of our governors. The governments of Europe have discovered education and in recent years have realized that you can bring up a generation to believe almost anything. Each of us has been moulded by the social system of which he forms a part. Our whole way of life, clothes, food, houses, family relationship, have all been taught us, and were we the inhabitants of India or New Guinea we should have been taught something different. It is only some sixty years since education became general in England and already the face of the country, and especially the towns has been changed. It is some fifteen years since Russia started to re-educate the nation to a completely new set of ideas and a new way of life. The remodelled state has taken shape and become comparatively stable. Among the other things that we are taught is submission to Government. We live in a continually growing net of regulations, and, as a nation, support an ever growing army of administrators to tell us what is right and proper. The ordinary citizen sees so much of one kind of Inspector or another, that he has almost ceased to think for himself. Thought is a bother ; and it is almost certain to be different from that of the Inspector—and therefore wrong. When to this established habit of submission to authority is added deliberate propaganda the state is almost unstable. The impulses of sympathy, imitation and suggestion, which are so important to the cohesion of society, may now prove its ruin. The State bases its appeals on all the more powerful impulses of man's nature, and the stronger the impulses appealed to by the leader the more violent the consequent acceptance of the suggestion. For example, what rendered the persecution of witches so violent was fear. No man knew that he might not be the next victim. It was the various instincts appealed to that made the Government propaganda in the Great War on the whole so successful.

In the days before 1914 war was considered as normal, and the terrible possibilities of a war between two European states not realized. Very few voices therefore were seriously raised against war in 1914, and those that were could hardly be heard among the shouts of mass excitement and the braying of Government propaganda and the vibrations of the emotions to which it appealed. There was of course fear, but that was not so effective in the very early days. During the period of the retreat from Mons when the newspaper placards said day after day " Glorious British retreat ", " Magnificent rearguard action ", it was plain anger, due to thwarted prestige, that flamed the strongest. It was only when the Germans approached Calais and were thus almost able to shell the south coast of England that fear was a vivid incentive. The next appeal was one based on a variation of the parental instinct : " Heroic *little* Belgium." Then sex, when a man was asked to defend his women from the outrages that had been inflicted on them in Belgium. Then personal self-respect with the famous slogan " What did you do in the Great War, Daddy ? " The posters on the sinking of the *Lusitania* were another series calculated to arouse indignation and fear. There were also such appeals to reason or semi-reason as that we were fighting a foe who would destroy liberty, or that if this war were victorious we should never be asked to fight again.

Recent events have shown how very explosive public feeling can be when a political idea is involved. It was only the firm determination of the British Government *not* to go to war that has prevented outbreaks of feeling over Abyssinia and Spain. A very small amount of government propaganda in favour of war would have armed the nation. It is interesting that those political parties have been most in favour of energetic action who on the whole are most opposed to war. The reason being that they have seen their principles threatened by the success of Fascist powers. Anger and the fighting spirit have kept up at a threat to any strong purpose.

We need then, if we are to abolish war, definite educational activity. We must not merely talk of the horrors of the next war, for a mere contemplation of horrors has never deterred a brave and determined man, but rather devote our efforts to forming (*a*) a belief in the impossibility of war, if not with all the world, at least with large parts of it, and (*b*) sentiments of active friendship with other nations, and (*c*) such common interests that there shall be the least possible excuse for friction.

This teaching will have to have the support of the Government. So long as the probability of war is kept before our minds by huge armament expenditure, so long as we are excited by air displays and military shows the true idea of peace cannot grow. The enormous power of organized propaganda cannot be resisted by individuals, it must be the articulate will of the whole group.

FOR DISCUSSION

1.—What do you think of the modern highly organized state?
   Would you prefer to have lived in a more individualistic age?
2.—" Oh, England is a pleasant place
      For them that's rich and high
      Oh, England is a cruel place
      For such poor men as I."
How far is that true to-day?

3.—Why do nations nowadays make so much more fuss about national status than they used to ?

4.—What *is* race ?   Why do some countries consider it so important ?

5.—Discuss the motive that lead certain nations to insist on a national language. E.g., the Welsh and Irish.

6.—What teaching on international problems would you give in school ?

7.—Discuss the complicated social effect of some other impulse, e.g., Nutrition.

BOOKS

R. HAGGART, *Nada the Lily*.   A story of the Zulu tyrant.

G. WALLAS, *The Great Society*.

WILLIAM JAMES, " The moral equivalent of War," in *Memories and Studies*.

A. A. MILNE, *Peace with Honour*.   A bitter indictment of modern militaristic ideas.

MASEFIELD, *The Faithful*.   The play is based on the Japanese story of the forty-seven Ronins—a study of the ethics of a military race.

The General.   A satire on the official military mind.

BERTRAND RUSSELL, *Which Way to Peace*.

FRANCIS WILLIAMS, *Plan for Peace*.

C. R. M. F. COUTTWELL, *A History of Peaceful Change in the Modern World*.

A. I. RICHARDS, *Hunger and Work in a Savage Tribe*.

TRAVEN, *The Death Ship*.   The adventures of a sailor who lost the proofs of his nationality.

75

CHAPTER VI

SEX AND PARENTAL INSTINCTS

"If he be not in love . . . there's no believing old signs; he brushes his hat o' mornings."

THE occupations connected with mating and the care of the young occupy a large part of the time and energy of the higher animals and man. Among the birds there is a period of courtship and mating, and then the partners devote their energies to nest building. The female lays eggs, and she and the male take turns at sitting on them. When the chicks are hatched they are fed by both birds, and later are taught to fly. If two families are reared in the summer this activity occupies the months from about April till July or August. In other animals varying amounts of parental care are given to the young. Sometimes the young are tended almost exclusively by the mother, as in the case of cats, and sometimes the father takes an almost equal share, as among sticklebacks, or birds.

In man, the long period of childhood and the continued unity of the family, even when the young are really able to fend for themselves, have made the function of parental care extremely important. In addition, the organization of society has caused considerable stress to be laid on the sex instinct. We have little means of knowing the conditions which accompany sexual relations in animals, and it seems likely that the ready satisfaction of sexual desires among some primitive peoples decreases the violence of the emotional accompaniments; but in a society which demands comparative chastity from its members, and prescribes a fairly long period of wooing before marriage, the emotional side of sex is very prominent.

Sex is one of the instincts which mature comparatively late in the development of the individual. For any real manifestation it must wait for physical maturity, but the first stirring of the instinct can be seen earlier. There is a period, about 18 months or 2 years of age, when a child's impulses can be seen with unusual clearness. The child is old enough to have power of action and not yet old enough to have learnt to modify his behaviour in accordance with social custom. At this age definite sexual interests appear. It is possible to watch flirtations between these tiny children and it is interesting to see how extraordinarily true to type they are. The girl coquette advances and retires, laughs, bats her lids and glances over her shoulder in a manner exactly like the film actress. The boy, as eager and less subtle, tries to catch her. This early expression of interest becomes much less marked as the child grows older. There are some children who are always susceptible to the other sex. All through their childhood the " interesting fact remains " that the playmate " was a little *boy* ", but this fact is treated so calmly by both children that it seems to be ignored. This apparent outward indifference to the sex relationship covers a growing understanding of what sex and marriage mean. There are many childish proposals of marriage—John, aged 8, writes to Mary aged seven : " Dear Mary, when we grow up will you marry me ? We will have three children, and we will ask Tom to be godfather because he is so good." Even where no such explicit declaration is made many children really love their playmates. They struggle with them, climb trees with them, play " desperate escaped criminals ", apparently without any sense of sexual differences. But they intend, with all the force of their being, to marry them at a later date. If, as generally happens, this intention is not fulfilled, the childish playmate retains a unique quality of romance that remains with the permanence of the unattainable ideal.

With the onset of adolescence this attitude changes. The child's mind is concerned above all with the body. Where the younger child, careless of his body except to delight in its efficiency, loved the mind of his playmate; the adolescent, often uncomfortable, has his attention

77

turned away from mere thought to physical changes and causes. There is the sudden interest in adornment, and the shyness that is due to an impulse of self-display that has not quite learned how to be most effective. Stevenson has described this change of attitude with the first oncoming of sexual maturity :

> The brooding boy, the sighing maid,
> Wholly fain and half afraid,
> Now meet along the hazel'd brook
> To pass and linger, pause and look.
>
> A year ago, and blithely paired,
> Their rough-and-tumble play they shared ;
> They kissed and quarrelled, laughed and cried,
> A year ago at Easter-tide.
>
> With bursting heart, with fiery face,
> She strove against him in the race ;
> He unabashed her garter saw,
> That now would touch her skirt with awe.
>
> And he to her a hero is,
> And sweeter she than primroses ;
> Their common silence dearer far
> Than nightingale and mavis are.

This period of adolescence, when the child is rapidly achieving sexual maturity, lasts from about 12 to 16 or 17 in girls and about 13 to 18 in boys. The age of development differs with individuals and with race or climate. It is, in England, rather a misfortune for a child to develop too early. Many boys suffer badly from a precocious development. Their voices break when their form-mates still have singing voices, their limbs grow too big, they have an incipient moustache. Such a boy is often bitterly ashamed of the development that no one has explained to him, and that he does not see repeated in his friends. It is then that a father or school master can give him real help. Girls, too, often need advice and help in understanding their development. Some schools give definite instructions—others do not, and presume that a mother has told her daughter all she needs to know. The modern mother is far less modest than her predecessor, and a girl's path is consequently easier. But every school should teach both boys and girls sufficient biology and human physiology for them to have a clear knowledge of the sexual and reproductive processes.

Adolescence is not only a physical process, it generally brings with it very considerable changes in outlook and thought. One of its earliest signs is an increased interest in dress. The grubby schoolboy, who has been the despair of his mother, now runs the risk of being late for school by spending so long brushing his hair. The girl dresses her hair for appearance instead of comfort. This new vanity differs from the child's pride · in his new shoes. The child will display itself to any audience ; the adolescent, though he fusses over his tie and pulls the corner of a coloured silk handkerchief from his pocket, blushes at any comment on his dress, and pretends that it is all nothing to him.

At the same time, particularly with girls, there is a marked change in the type of literature read. Novels, especially those of hopeless love, become the favourite matter. Modern descendants of *Coming Thro' the Rye* move to tears and raptures. Poetry, too, begins to be appreciated for its own sake. This is only natural as such a large part of our best poetry is either definitely erotic or contains erotic similes. The youth explores the Bible and is suddenly delighted by the magnificent sensuousness of the *Song of Solomon*. Even the hardened athlete may be seen stuffing a Swinburne into his pocket, or putting Browning under the sofa cushions when suddenly disturbed.

A new love of literature is not the only mental activity involved in this renaissance. The developing sex instinct seems to liberate a large amount of energy, part of which is expended in intellectual activity. Adolescence is the period of religious doubts and conversions. The Anglican Church has recognized this and has, therefore, made the the age of 14–16 the normal age for confirmation, when religious and moral teaching of a certain sort is given.

At about this age also, children begin to feel an increased sense of personal responsibility ; and many treat the matter of their careers very seriously, supposing they are enjoying an education which allows them to remain so long undecided. Many schools, in consequence, make special provision for specialization beginning about this age.

Towards the end of adolescence, interest in politics develops, and the young politician becomes an ardent Socialist, or a devoted Tory of the extreme Right Wing. Moderation has no meaning for him, and in the first flush of excitement he is willing to die, and does die daily in his day dreams, at the head of his victorious partisans.

This type of adolescent is, of course, not universal, and some people pass through the period tranquilly, the poorer, probably, for not having experienced its anguish and excitements.

In others of less intellectual power the development and manifestation of the sex impulse is more direct. First for the girl a period of adoration of some slightly older girl or woman (the period, this, of " grand passions "), and then the girl gets a " boy ", and the period of courting begins in play or earnest. So with men—the youth worships some hero of his own sex—a footballer or a prize fighter, and then is ready in the normal course to fall in love with one of the opposite sex.

But because much of value is acquired in the period of adolescence in cases when the sex instinct, baulked of its natural outlet, lends energy to various forms of intellectual activity ; and because once a girl or boy has really fallen in love it is hard to keep his or her attention on other subjects ; schools definitely try to delay the full development of the sex instinct as long as possible. To this end they make the children play games (since physical exercise drains off energy which would be directed to other channels) and set up ideals of the strenuous life which are directly opposed to the early development of sex relations. Except in co-education schools, social relations between boys and girls—particularly at boarding-schools—are discouraged. This policy of segregation and strenuous physical exertion is carried on in some universities and most training colleges and the advisability of the policy forms one of the chief arguments against co-education.

It is claimed by a certain type of psychologist that nearly all the abnormalities of childhood are due to unsatisfied sexual curiosity ; and the treatment proposed is to give the child the information that he is supposed to be in need of. In the published accounts of cases it seems very doubtful if the child's difficulties were really due to this cause, or if the treatment were very successful. There is no doubt whatever that many children, quite young as well as adolescents, suffer from a guilty curiosity that is simply due to ignorance and the hush-hush attitude of their parents. The extreme ignorance of the Victorian girl of marriageable age was amazing and pathetic. It hardly ever exists to-day. A child in a family first starts asking questions about the birth of babies when he is 2 to 4 years old. He is then mainly interested in the mother's part, and will ask very intelligent questions. To answer him is right and proper ; and a child so answered shows no surprise or shock. It is a mistake to keep on harping on the subject, or to keep referring to it all through the mother's pregnancy for the next baby. Interest in the father's part of the process comes later. Some children of 8 or 9 are deeply interested in the information, and seem delighted to know it. Others appear slightly embarrassed. The information may be given too early or late, and is much more difficult to explain to the child than the mother's share, which he seems to grasp at once ; in some cases he even appears to know it without any telling. If there is proper teaching in school, or the child is provided with proper books of reference, many of the troubles of adolescence vanish. So many girls, who are quite ignorant of the causes or signs of pregnancy, imagine that they are going to have a baby and worry themselves almost ill. Other children, equally causelessly, imagine that they have suffered some mutilation or contracted some disease. If there is no adequate teaching in school and the parents feel incompetent, it is often a good plan to send an adolescent child round to the family doctor for a talk and good advice. They usually greatly appreciate this opportunity of saying what is in their minds.

Most people experience at least one love affair and learn for themselves the joys of a measure of sex satisfaction. Sex experiences are certainly a subject on which people love to dwell. As has been said, a large part of our poetry is concerned with this sexual love ; it enters in one form or another into most novels ; hardly a play or a film is quite complete without some love element ; and, moreover, it forms the basis of a considerable part of our thoughts.

Hence arises the problem for the unmarried woman. She is never allowed, under our moral code, full satisfaction for a very important part of her nature, one which is continually being stimulated by events around her. Occasionally a woman in this situation manages to develop into the perfect aunt, contented in her own sphere and generously willing to share in the joys of others, retaining a love for children, and behaving naturally and pleasantly in the company of men. Others develop less happily. They may take to themselves women friends whom they love with the devotion they would have given to a male lover. Others again, try to turn their backs on thoughts of sex and may grow to dislike men, find babies intolerable, and regard the courting of youths and maidens as disgusting. Others again, give to lap-dogs or pets the loving care they would have given normally to children.

The young unmarried woman who has not yet become the old maid has her own troubles. The thought of sex in one form or another is often a very persistent one and invades her day and night dreams in a way which she not infrequently regards as wicked, or, at least, degrading. In addition to this she is often subject to recurrent fits of sex excitement, which, though not apparently traceable to any definite experience, are strong and most disturbing. The easiest remedy for such a state is a dance or a social evening ; but if she is one of the many thousands of women, particularly teachers, who live in lodgings in towns where they have few friends, physical exercise is perhaps the best palliative. A sharp walk, a folk dance class, and vigorous exercise ending in a cold bath, are all ways of restoring a more settled state of mind.

The sex instinct, when it passes beyond mere lust, is generally accompanied by feelings of tender care for its object. There is a stage in a courtship when the lover becomes very solicitous about the physical welfare of his beloved.

> A pity beyond all telling
> Is hid in the heart of love:
> The folk that are buying and selling
> The clouds in their journey above,
> The cold wet winds ever blowing
> And the shadowy hazel grove
> Where the mouse-grey waters are flowing,
> Threaten the head that I love.[1]

This is normally followed after marriage by affectionate care and reciprocal tenderness. Occasionally, however, a perversion appears and sex excitement becomes connected with tendencies to cruelty. The part played by pain and violence in sex matters is responsible for the horse-whipping and other such outrages which occur in certain novels of passion, and for the pleasant thrill which one may feel when reading such accounts.[2] It is also in part responsible for the charm of certain austerities which were commonplaces in mediæval life, and which, though practised in secret, still in some cases exist to-day.

The parental instinct, like the sexual, is not fully developed till maturity, and then it needs the actual presence of a child to call it forth in its full force. But it is manifested in a rudimentary form early in life. Little girls love their dolls. Many girls often find the greatest pleasure in taking a baby out for a walk. In schools, lessons on the care of babies are always popular with the older children. For women, married or unmarried, the attraction of babies is very strong, though, of course, it varies with individuals. Some people find themselves more attracted to little babies, others do not like children till these have reached a certain age. To men, many of whom have this instinct strongly, the child from two years old or so is most charming.

The development of the parental instinct has had very

---

[1] Yeats' *Poems, The Pity of Love.* Cf. also *Ungrounded fears torment the lover.*—Wordsworth.

[2] Cf. *The Sheik, The Knave of Diamonds,* and many other popular novels Violence in one form or another regularly occurs in the writings of E. M. Dell.

considerable effects. This is especially so in man where the period of dependence is longest. If the young have to fend for themselves immediately at birth they need to be born with their reactions to the environment well defined and sufficiently definite to be immediately serviceable. The young of many insects and crustaceans, receive no parental care and can look after themselves at once. There is, consequently, less possibility of learning by experience. Moreover, if they are not in association with their parents they will learn only from their own individual experience. There will thus be no opportunity for succeeding generations of the species to build up a body of traditional experience, and they will lack one of the most indispensable conditions of progress.

Man, who is born helpless, has abundant opportunities of acquiring the modes of behaviour which are most completely in harmony with his surroundings. Through his long association with his parents he becomes inheritor of the mass of knowledge and ways of thought and feeling, which make up our civilization. The increasing importance of this period of dependence is shown by the way in which it has lengthened as man has become more civilized, as well as by the fact that it is longest for the most highly educated members of the community.

As soon as a child begins to earn its living it is forced to acquire a fixed set of habits, and to perfect itself in some more or less routine task. This for the average person means a cessation of that freedom of thought and a loss of that plasticity of mind which make education possible. Even in the rare cases where this does not happen, the demands of work make such heavy inroads on time and energy that there is comparatively little of either available for private investigation.

In consequence, where workers are expected also to add to the world's knowledge—as in the case of university lecturers—the hours of teaching are cut down to a point which will permit of individual research.

Thus, children who are going to be doctors, teachers, engineers, lawyers, and so on, are kept dependent for a comparatively long period, about a third or quarter of their lives. During this time they are supported by the labour of others, either directly or in the form of stored wealth, and allowed to acquire the skill which they will need later.

The length of the period is determined by two things, the amount of knowledge to be acquired, and the fact that much of it *can* only be acquired when the mind is fairly mature. It is useless to expect a child to study philosophy. The problems with which it is concerned are entirely beyond his world of thought, and, so long as a nation thinks it needs philosophers and their like, so long must it maintain students comparatively free from the need to earn their living up to the age of 22 or thereabouts. Similar arguments justify the maintenance of children at secondary schools, or, for that matter, even at primary ones. Children of five can be, and have been, employed in industry, but the practice has been found to be not only inhuman but uneconomical, since under such a system the race is deprived of citizens equipped with the social heritage acquired during a long dependent period.

There is a modern claim that sex and reproduction, being in essence two different things, should be separate in practice : and that marriage should not be " First, for the procreation of children, to be brought up in the fear and nurture of the Lord . . ." but rather that the pleasures of sexual intercourse should be enjoyed for themselves without being necessarily followed by offspring. The modern spread of knowledge has made this point of view tenable, but how far it is psychologically sound it is difficult to say. If man and the animals are as closely akin as some researches seem to suggest, the unnatural division in man of functions that are naturally linked may seem unwise. On the other hand, no modern woman would consent to go back to the Victorian ideal of a baby a year. Perhaps the solution is the common one of moderation ; man should use his knowledge rather to improve on the arrangements of nature than to deny them. This is seen very clearly in the strain that childlessness imposes on most marriages ; and in a country such as Ceylon, where there are practically no children, as they all have to be sent home quite young because of the climate, the effects on the domestic life of the European residents is usually deplorable. On the whole, too, children are desired. It is an economic rather than a psychological difficulty that suggests the limitation or complete refusal of a family. Both sex and the parental instinct extend their effects beyond their direct objects and have considerable effects in our social life. In a trivial way we can see their power on the covers of our magazines and the posters of our hoardings. The commonest magazine cover is the picture of a pretty girl, and the next commonest, especially on those intended to appeal to women, is a bonny baby. So, too, soap and cocoa, whisky and cornflour, a new play or novel, try to catch our attention by representing young women or children. Our interest is caught by the natural stimulant to an instinct, and even the slight satisfaction to the instinct given by the picture produces a feeling of pleasure, which attaches in thought to the object advertised. In a similar way there are few parts of a newspaper so soothing to many a tired woman as the " woman's page ". The insistence on dress, with the implication of the importance of sex relations, gratifies an instinct without shocking a sense of the proprieties.

In more serious matters, too, we can see the effects of these instincts. The tendency to protect or care for the young extends itself to any small or helpless thing, and outbursts of moral indignation greet the maltreatment of animals and helpless persons. Much capital was made in the last War out of the comparative sizes of Belgium and Germany. *Punch's* cartoons represented Belgium as a boy resisting the attacks of a grown man. So, too, the tendency to protect his wife will make a man furious at any outrage to a woman. This instinctive reaction partly accounts for the ideals of chivalry. This is one of the reasons why this virtue is characteristic of the adolescent rather than the small boy.

Our feelings towards such a brigand as Robin Hood are due to the causes described above. He wins our instinctive sympathy because he championed the poor against the rich, the weak against the strong, and in all cases defended women against aggressors. Consequently, he has become a member of the school pantheon along with such " gentlemen adventurers " as Drake, Dick

86

SEX AND PARENTAL INSTINCTS

Turpin, and Richard Lion Heart, whose morals, however questionable in some respects, satisfy the elementary code we have described. Even in our own day, we have a certain respect for the good brigand. The "cat burglar", so long as he confines his attention to Park Lane and Mayfair, is not without his attractions. Cinema films illustrate the same tendency. We see many lawless deeds done by Wild West heroes, but few acts of positive cruelty.

Neither the sex nor the paternal instinct operates alone. In each case many other tendencies co-operate in attaining the aims which they set. Sexual jealousy will provoke the most violent anger, and so, as has been said above, will a slight to one's own child. Self-assertion and submission are also closely connected with them, and so is fear—for the beloved object, though both sex and parental instincts will inhibit fear for personal safety if the object of the instinct is in danger.

FOR DISCUSSION

1.—Describe, as much as possible from your own observation, the mental changes of adolescence.
2.—Give a list of your favourite books, stating the ages at which you liked them.
3.—Discuss the merits of co-education.
4.—Discuss the problems raised by a falling population.
5.—If society provides the money for a man's education, what rights has it to his services when his education is completed?
6.—Consider and try to account for the popularity of Greta Garbo and Shirley Temple.
7.—How far is it right to say (with **Prof.** McDougall) that the Parental Instinct is the root of all morality?
8.—Discuss the different standards suggested by a comparison of Gilbert and Sullivan's *Patience*, Tennyson's *Princess*, and Shaw's *Candida*.

BOOKS

For types and phases of love:
ROBERT BROWNING, *Porphyria's Lover ; The Statue and the Bust ; By the Fire-side.*
MARLOWE, *Hero and Leander.*
EDMUND SPENSER, *Epithalamion.*
SHAKESPEARE, *Sonnets, Romeo and Juliet.*
MASEFIELD, *The Daffodil Fields.*
For a discussion of some problems of marriage:
G. B. SHAW, *Getting Married ; Pygmalion* (the epilogue).

MAY SINCLAIR, *Life and Death of Harriett Freen.* ⎫ Problems of sex
ROSE MACAULAY, *Dangerous Ages.*   ⎬ adjustment in
                                                    ⎭   women

MELANIE KLEIN, *Psycho-Analysis of Children.*

SUSAN ISAACS, *Social Development of Young Children.*

K. DE SCHWEINITZ, *How a Baby is Born.* A very good book for children.

W. McDOUGALL, *Character and the Conduct of Life.* A surprising variety of good advice.

CHAPTER VII

CONSTRUCTION, BEAUTY AND ACQUISITION

" What make you here ? "
" Nothing, Sir. I am not taught to make anything."
" What mar you, then ? "

WE have taken some of the main instincts and shown the way in which they affect thought and social life. In this chapter some tendencies will be discussed which are of less importance than those already described, but which yet play a large part in the lives of many people. If an instinct is defined as an innate tendency to perceive certain objects, to experience a certain emotion and to act in a certain way, the tendencies to construct and to acquire can hardly be called instincts. They are innate tendencies, but they are not directed to specific objects, and no special emotion seems to be connected with them. However, their exact status is not so important as the fact that they exist and operate in definite ways.

The tendency to make or construct things of use or beauty occurs among the animals, particularly among birds, and is generally found in the service of some other instinct. Birds build nests for their eggs and their young, the caddis worm protects itself with its case, but the bower bird seems to construct its arbours purely for pleasure, if we may believe the story that it decks the moss in front with bright flowers and removes them when they are withered ; yet even here an instinct seems indirectly to be served, for the birds do their courting in the arbours, building their nests elsewhere.

Among men this tendency was no doubt originally connected strictly with the needs of life. Primitive man made shelters to protect himself from the weather, skin wrappings for warmth or armour, weapons for war or hunting, simple utensils for domestic needs, and perhaps an ornament to make himself attractive in the eyes of, the other sex, or to impress his fellows with the importance of his position as chieftain or priest.

With a life of increasing complexity, men find less direct expression for this tendency to construct in their every-day work. Mass production has led to specialization of labour. A man spends his days making grooves in wooden frames, or buttons, or seaming trousers or putting rims on saucers, and all this probably by the aid of a machine, instead of, as formerly, constructing a whole house or garment or utensil designed by himself and fashioned to his own purposes. But the tendency to construct satisfies itself in other ways—part of the joy of a bicycle to a youth is the continual reconstruction necessary for its mainten-ance. The fretwork enthusiast pursues his hobby for the joy of making something, rather than because he wants the thing he makes—and the same is true of the elaborate embroideries in wool of the last century.

Among modern men the strength of the constructive tendency varies greatly, partly by natural endowment, partly through the influence of environment ; but where it is strong it can be one of the greatest pleasures of life, especially as it is closely intertwined with æsthetic appre-ciation. In a simple stage of society a man constructs mainly for his own use, and, in consequence, his work is done to the best of his ability. It is no good making oneself a pair of boots of bad materials or with imperfect workmanship.

Moreover, the tendency to make the object beautiful as well as useful, is nearly always present. There is a primitive appreciation of a quality which may be called " prettiness ", which develops at an early age. The Binet tests require a child of four to be able to tell which of two faces (one obviously ugly) is the prettier ; many quite small children select and show their appreciation of " pretty " colours—even if their taste does not always agree with ours. The craftsman, therefore, making an object for his own use, makes it " pretty " to the best of this ability, in just the same way that he makes it useful, and there is no real opposition between these two terms in a simple state of life. This simple taste is good, as one can see from peasant costumes and pottery, or from the bowls which have come down to us from the neolithic age.

The craftsman fell into disrepute when the world went mad over the new power and precision of machinery, which could multiply ornament so rapidly that it was added simply for its own sake, whether it suited the article to which it was added or not. The elaborate machine-made wood carving which encrusts the overmantels and furniture of the 1880's and 1890's, and which serves no useful or artistic purpose, is a good example of this kind of art. Morris and Ruskin were the pioneers of the movement which was necessary to revive appreciation of the beauty of the hand-made article and of the dignity of the craftsman who made it. By this time their doctrine is established. Most people prefer hand-woven materials and hand-embroidered dresses, hand-carved furniture and fine cut glass to the machine-made articles. Our difficulty is that we cannot afford them.

We have also learnt to respect the craftsman. In a slave-owning society manual work was certain to be felt as degrading. Plato, for example, declares that the mechanic is rightly excluded from the franchise because his occupation warps his mind just as it does his body. This prejudice against manual labour died hard. It is not even quite dead in some cases to-day [1]—but, theoretically at all events, a large part of the populace rejects it. In towns where there is more intellectual than industrial activity, and the bulk of the populace is comfortably off, though not rich, handicrafts and manual labour are common hobbies and are much respected. In Oxford it is no uncommon thing for a professor to practise wood carving as a hobby, and not a few undergraduates may be seen in vacation painting the front railings of their houses. In Germany economic conditions have forced the student to turn manual labourer in his vacations and the " work student " is becoming a common figure.

[1] e.g., Amateur rowing clubs.

This has been the practice for some years in Canada and U.S.A.

Once the prejudice against manual labour is removed, it is possible to appreciate its pleasures. For many people, under proper conditions, there is no more delightful occupation. The whole process is fraught with a strong sense of life and activity : the craftsman imagines the thing he is going to make, he plans and devises, shaping his idea to fit his materials ; then he lays his hand to the work and sees, bit by bit, his idea take external form ; when it is done he contemplates it and sees—like God— that " it is good ".

It is hard to imagine a more perfect cycle of activity than the successful making of even a simple object ; and, unlike some pleasures, this brings no unpleasant after-effects ; no headaches, and no regrets. But this perfect activity is only possible if circumstances are propitious. In the first place the worker must feel that he is an inventor as well as an executor. It is not interesting to work to the directions of another if one feels competent to work alone. The case is different while one is learning. One rather likes being asked to make, for example, a silk dressing-gown, but half the pleasure would be gone if one were supplied with the silk and the pattern by which it was to be cut out ; and one would probably refuse the commission, if the amount, pattern and colour of the embroidery were also specified. We enjoy the challenge to our ingenuity contained in the problem to be solved quite as much as we enjoy the actual work.

Too often in schools this fact is neglected. The teacher is so anxious that the children should make their " wall tidies ", for example, accurately, that she prescribes each step as carefully as if they were employees of Ford's ; and, though she may show them the finished article, she often forgets to allow them to make their own plans for carrying out the work. If the children want to make the article, they will rejoice to have to plan and adapt it for themselves, and will be ready enough to ask the necessary help in the doing of it ; unless they are allowed to feel personal power in the making, they lose that pleasure which would be the incentive to further efforts.

Secondly, good work cannot be done in a hurry, and working to time destroys the pleasure even of the most attractive job. The worker must, therefore, be allowed to work at his own pace, which is not the same for all people. Nor is the method of work the same with all. One need go no further afield than the tasks of daily life, to be convinced of this. If you and your friend are cutting out a frock, or doing a piece of carpentry, or papering a room, differences of method and speed at once become obvious. One method may, objectively, be better than the other, but each worker prefers his own, and works better if allowed to use it. So small a matter as the way paste is put on to a strip of wall-paper before hanging it may disclose fundamental differences of procedure. For enjoyment the craftsman must have his own methods of work. He may be shown better ones and adopt them, but then they become part of himself and are modified to fit his own needs. When he is forced to work at a pace or in a manner which is felt to be alien, he becomes a slave once more. Many of the modern theories of industry involve a systematization and exact timing of operations ; these systems, when properly applied, do undoubtedly increase output, and are usually accompanied by a rise in wages and a shortening of the hours of work. Yet they are often met by the most determined opposition from the workers, who feel their old pride of work slipping from them and all pleasure to be taken from it.

Lastly, to obtain satisfaction, a man needs to make a whole thing. The crown of craftsmanship is the contemplation of the finished article. In modern industry this is too frequently denied. The work has been subdivided so that each worker performs one small part of the task and, in consequence, never has the opportunity of enjoying the total result. The matter is, of course, rather different, when several people each make one thing to be used in some larger whole which they will construct ; when, for instance, in school, one child makes a hut, another dresses a doll and the third constructs a palm tree, all to be used in an illustration of Indian life. It is probable that, when the whole model is done, each child will gaze with peculiar affection at his own contribution, but he will really achieve a double pleasure from this mode of work—the joy of making his own contribution, and the pleasure of seeing it used in a larger whole.

The craftsman, then, who works in his own way, produces an article which seems to him good, i.e., it possesses the qualities of usefulness and beauty. This is the earliest form of art and the one which is most popular with children. In a school which does both fine art and handicrafts, given comparable teaching, the crafts are the more popular.

Constructive activity has a far larger part than this to play in a child's development. Dr. Charlotte Bühler has pointed out that constructive power is one of the best indications of a child's development, and one of the best aids to the process. A very little child can make nothing : a child deprived of opportunities for constructive play is late in learning the ideas we associate with " work ", and is very difficult to instruct in school. If he is to be made teachable he must be given the experience of construction that he has lacked at home. It is interesting to study the development of constructive power in children. The simplest is that belonging to the type of building with bricks. From about 18 months a child will pile bricks together and enjoy both the building and the resulting crash. The improvement of the activity takes place in many ways.

(1) The child's hand becomes steadier and his power of accurate placing increases. This is a definite sign of mental growth. Mentally defective children are conspicuous for their poor muscular control.

(2) The structure built begins to have meaning. It is not just a pile of bricks, it is " my house ", " a garage " or " the king's castle '.

(3) The construction becomes more complex. There are various rooms to the house, or gates to the castle.

(4) Various processes are involved. The child begins to experiment with methods of roofing spaces or of building doorways.

Just as the activity becomes more complex so does its importance for the child increase. Charlotte Bühler would stress the conception of the "job", the imagination of something to be done and the carrying out of the plan. This is to a certain extent true, but so many childish constructions run on from one thing to another that the task has no well defined limits and no natural end. More important is the outlet for the imagination that such construction gives. This will be discussed in another chapter.

Naturally constructive work gives a training in manual skill. The child learns to use his hands, and not only to use but to trust them. There are so many people—fewer in this generation than the last—who are incompetent in manual activities, and fear them in consequence. They represent, in many cases, the results of a home where manual activities had no place. This was particularly the fate of boys of the richer classes under the educational ideas of the last century.

The self-confidence that construction gives extends farther than manual work. Power to do anything increases a child's self-respect, and therefore his value to himself and others. It is for this reason that constructional work has in part been substituted for academic with those children who learn slowly and with distaste from books.

For the adult there is a further moral gain in the pursuit of some skilled craft. The craftsman has to enter into a special relation with his material. He must subdue himself to it—spiritually—so that he may control it in his turn. The result is that the skilled craftsman is one of the best members of society. Taken as a class they seem to possess all the virtues. They are dignified, self-respecting, kind, patient, honest. They are not on the whole very articulate. They are not always skilled in the use of words, so that those who produce theories of the state and education take a long time to discover their superlative merits. But one has only to get to know them, whether they are miners or jewellers, to realize that the training they have undergone has produced virtues and abilities that an academic education in many cases strikingly fails to provide.

The craftsman is the forerunner of the pure artist. When possessions multiply and life begins to be stable and wealthy, we find fine art arising by the side of applied. In a civilization such as that in Crete about 1400 B.C., we find beautiful drinking bowls, inlaid swords, jewellery, statues of the gods, and coloured frescoes. These frescoes represent birds or flying fish, figures of kings or pictures of scenes in the country, or bull fights in the palace arena. This art of the frescoes has severed itself from strict utility and has begun to take an independent position. This has happened with each civilization in turn, and in certain of them, e.g., in that of Western Europe to-day, fine art is divorced from the crafts, and, on the whole, considers itself superior to them. It is doubtful whether fine art gains by this separation. It certainly is no gainer by the theorists who talk of " art for art's sake ", or believe Whistler's doctrine—forced on him by the cold reception his pictures received—that the artist alone is concerned with a work of art, and that the praise of the public— if given—is a mere impertinence.

When art is closely connected with crafts and decoration, two main characteristics appear in it, the quality of prettiness mentioned above, and technical perfection. In fine art there is room for a third element—meaning. We can see all these elements in such a picture as the Sistine Madonna. The figures, colouring and composition are all pleasing ; the technique is so good that we can see what the artist meant us to see in drapery and texture ; and the idea behind it, the meaning, the conception of beautiful and pure motherhood is ennobling. Different artists, or schools of artists, excel in different elements. The rich colours in Titian's " Bacchus and Ariadne " are delightful, the Dutch painters were masters of the art of suggesting textures and surfaces, and many of the primitive painters, e.g., Giotto, have a nobleness of conception which is lacking in more finished painters.

These qualities can be brought out by contrasting good and bad art which possess somewhat the same qualities. Leonardo's " Mona Lisa ", set beside a chocolate box lady, does not so much excel in beauty of colour or feature, as in meaning. Aubrey Beardsley's illustrations to *Salome* are technically almost perfect—certainly the equal of Dürer's drawings, yet their sensual unhealthiness disgusts the majority of normal people. Van Eyck's portrait of Arnolfini of Lucca cannot match with Velasquez' " Venus " for beauty, though the former may be technically the equal of the latter.

The simplest form of the appreciation of a work of art is to find it " pretty ". This is what a child does, and what the majority of unsophisticated adults do. Although the theories and practices of many modern artists seem to discredit this " prettiness ", to cut this element out of art is to strike at the very root of the æsthetic experience. " Prettiness " is not all, and to give it too great importance is to stultify art, but it is the fundamental experience to which the others are added. The other two elements are appreciated according to circumstances. A fellow-craftsman can most easily appreciate the qualities of construction and appraise the success of the result because he knows the difficulties. To achieve this appreciation fully we must ourselves be practitioners—even if in a humble way—of the same art. This was the method of appreciation employed by Robert Browning. The comprehension of meaning depends on the range of our own experience. Fully to appreciate a work of art we must ourselves to some extent have lived through the experience portrayed ; what is clear to one is a riddle to another, and our likes and dislikes are largely influenced by our emotional knowledge. These latter types of appreciation, therefore, are only in a very limited degree available to the child.

The appreciation of " prettiness " is largely inarticulate. If we stand under beech trees on a fine day in October, and look at the leaves against the sky and the tree trunk, and see the leaves falling, we may be filled by a wave of emotion at the beauty of the sight. We expand ourselves to it and try in every way to bring ourselves into closer contact with it, but the appreciation is not articulate. If we say anything, it is simply " How lovely ! " We do not, until after, analyse our experience. The same thing happens with art—we appreciate long before we can make our appreciation analytic. The art critic is, therefore, a late and bastard product of art. He is not a craftsman, and he is not the simple appreciator. He goes round telling us *why* we like what we do like, and because he can say least about the most fundamental and important thing in art—sheer beauty—he is always trying to turn us into antiquarians or vorticists, or to thrill us with reproductions of revolting negro Venuses. About these things he can talk—they need explanation or defence. He is interesting ; archæology is a fascinating subject, and the vagaries of the human mind excellent psychological matter ; but he does not bring us any nearer to real appreciation. He only makes us articulate and teaches us phrases. At his best he explains the historical development of an artist and his place in the movements of his time, or the conditions under which his technique developed. Here he is useful, but he is useful as a historian and not as a critic.

This applies very strongly in schools. If we are going to give children æsthetic appreciation it must be real and not merely verbal. They must be presented with objects of beauty, pictures, poems, music, and must be allowed to enjoy them. For this simple enjoyment more things are necessary than every teacher can command. The poems must be well read, the pictures well hung, the music well played. There must be opportunities for repetition—familiarity is a great aid to love—and reflection ; there must be no dense wall of ignorance to block the view. When all this has been achieved, the work of art—if it is itself good—can be left to speak for itself, and make its own appeal. If anything further is needed, it is best achieved by the natural road of personal effort. The writing of a poem teaches more about poetic structure than any number of exhortations to "observe the pathos of this line ". Once the children have begun to write their own poems they have a basis to work from. They know what kind of thing the poet wanted to do, and they look to see how he did it. All the talk of the critics, which before was empty, now takes on meaning. Such dry subjects as the rhyme schemes of stanzas acquire importance, and rhythm with all its variations and niceties becomes a province of wonder. So in art ; to start to paint is to find the gates of appreciation opening—so in drama ; the simplest form-room play if taken intelligently can teach us more about Shakespeare than one could ever learn without it.

Towards the third element, the apprehension of meaning, we can do less. No school explanation of the deadly weariness of a town will ever make children, who have not felt the emotion, fully enter into the spirit of the *Lake Isle of Innisfree*, nor will any talk bring home to boys of ten or eleven the significance of Shelley's *Ode to Night*. This difficulty can be met by giving children works of art which express ideas with which they may be supposed to be familiar, and leaving the rest till time has instructed them. This familiarity may be in imagination as well as fact. Children are imaginatively familiar with fairies, with idyllic love stories of princes and princesses, with talking beasts and with heroic adventures of knights, although these things have never come within their actual experience.

Acquisition is another tendency which appears sporadically in animals, and, to a far greater extent, among men. Squirrels and other animals hoard nuts, ants and bees lay in stores, and jackdaws will pick up bright objects which are of no use to them. This acquisitive tendency often appears in children, who collect cigarette cards, postcards, stamps, marbles or bright stones, without having any real use for the collection, or even imagining a use. This collecting tendency becomes in some men the passion of their lives—especially when it is joined with the competitive spirit or the desire for power. It generally allies itself with some other aim ; they are scientists and collect birds, insects or beetles to further the growth of knowledge ; they love art and collect prints or pictures, which they keep in portfolios or in rooms they seldom visit ; they desire the power of wealth and collect golden sovereigns or bank script. They are even imperialists, like Cecil Rhodes, and collect provinces. It is not uncommon to find the collecting tendency given a rational explanation. A man says he is anxious for wealth because he wishes to be secure from poverty ; yet he continues to amass money long after all danger of want or even inconvenience is removed. Another collector says he hunts moths in the interests of science, and keeps his collection shut up where no one but himself can see it.[1] The inadequacy of the reason given to explain the action shows the true instinctive tendency lying behind it.

It seems likely that the acquisitive tendency was first organized, as were the instincts, to meet a definite need. When man developed from his prehuman ancestors he began to use tools. He hunted, fought, and later kept flocks or tilled the ground. For all these purposes he needed implements, and it would be natural for each man to have his own, fitted to his strength and grasp. If they were weapons of war on which his life depended, he would himself look to their security. Thus, even while many things, such as houses or canoes, were common property, it would be natural for a man to own his small personal belongings. It is to these, even to-day, that we cling most strongly. Many people do not much mind not owning the house they live in—so long as the landlord keeps it in decent repair—but to have no private property in one's fountain pen or wrist watch would be very trying.

The accumulation of property beyond these simple needs probably took place under the influence of two tendencies. Possession both gave and showed power, so that the chief was rich when he was chosen and used his chieftaincy to become richer. Property is also a defence, thus the anxious seek to shield themselves behind a rampart of wealth.

These two motives influence acquisition to-day very strongly. Great wealth gives great power over our fellow human beings, moderate wealth gives certain powers, as over employees. But wealth is even more prized for the feeling of security that it brings. To know that, come what may, one has £300 a year certain, relieves one from a thousand carking anxieties. Moreover, even this amount of money means an increase in personal power. One is freer of space—one can travel ; freer of time—one can delegate to others the tasks that hinder progress. From this point of view moderate acquisition is of social advan-

[1] For a treatment of this tendency from many aspects, see Galsworthy's *Forsyte Saga*.

tage. It enables the cleverer men, those who can manage to acquire enough, to live in a way which gives greater scope for their special talents.

On the other hand, private property has frequently been the object of attack. Plato in his ideal state abolished it as he abolished the family [1]; devout men of religion take vows of poverty ; a few extreme communists dream of a society as nearly as possible without private ownership. Yet it is asserted that children brought up in institutions where they have nothing of their own suffer from the lack, and it is hard for most people to envisage a happy life without some private possessions. Those who have had the experience of living for some months or years in trunks, or without a fixed abode wherein to keep their treasured possessions, know how worrying continual rebuffs to the acquisitive tendency can be. Moreover, it has happened that the accumulation of large stores of wealth in private hands and the desire for further possessions have led to the production of many of the finest works of art we possess. The Renaissance Popes were great patrons of art and more concerned about gold buttons for their copes than about points of doctrine. Their patronage did much to encourage and secure the great art produced in the Renaissance Age. To-day art is in a different position and looks to public bodies for support rather than to private patrons. This certainly makes the products of art more accessible to the people at large ; whether it makes for the greater happiness of the artist or the merit of his work is uncertain.

From the standpoint of sociology it is necessary to distinguish beneficial from harmful acquisition, and the dividing line seems to lie where possession carries with it rights, which may be misused, over the lives and liberties of others. In the ownership of purely personal possessions there is not harm but good. For our health and comfort we need to own our tools and those things of which we make daily use ; some proportion of the things we make ; and, in addition, certain unnecessary things that are our toys. Grown-ups as well as children need them, and just as Tommy cannot reach the full height

[1] *The Republic.*

of felicity without a horse and cart to play with, so his father lacks complete happiness if he has not a wireless set for the same purpose.

FOR DISCUSSION

1.—What part should handwork play in education ? Sketch what you consider the principles governing the best methods of teaching it.
2.—What are the economic problems involved in a general return to craft production ?
3.—By what means can modern mechanical production be made less harmful for the worker ?
4.—Discuss the difference between school " handwork " and learning a skilled craft.
5.—What are the earliest signs of æsthetic activity or appreciation in children ? Are they against or in accord with the theory given in the book ?
6.—Discuss means by which æsthetic appreciation can be inculcated in schools.
7.—Suggest any explanation you can of the judgment of " beauty ".
8.—Apply to literature the remarks about painting in our chapter.
9.—What is the difference between beauty in nature and in art ?
10.—What are the sociological objections and advantages in the accumulation of property ?
11.—Describe any examples you have observed in yourself or others of the acquisitive tendency, stating the age of development, the direction of the tendency, and the alleged reasons for it.
12.—By what means would you attempt to educate the acquisitive tendency in children ?
13.—What is your opinion of the " appreciation " lesson in literature ? Describe such a lesson, showing its advantages and weaknesses.
14.—Is there a place in the school syllabuses for art (e.g., pictures, literature and music) which is not fully understood by the children ? If so, show how you would present such art to the children.
15.—A modern critic avers that there is no such thing as beauty ; but that we can only describe the physical effects of sound, colour, etc., in ourselves. Discuss this.
16.—Make a record of the colours that the children you know prefer. (You might experiment with coloured pieces of material and ask them to choose the prettiest.) Observe the stage when children begin to recognize and name shapes.
17.—Why do we take pleasure in certain designs ? Describe a design for wall paper or printed silk, or a book plate which particularly pleases you and say what element in it gives you pleasure.
18.—Justify the place of the art critic in modern society.

BEAUTY AND ACQUISITION

BOOKS

R. H. TAWNEY, *The Acquisitive Society.* An attack on modern capitalist society.

G. D. H. COLE, *Labour in the Commonwealth.* A general discussion of labour problems from a socialist's standpoint. *Guild Socialism Restated.* A suggested reorganization of industry that would place control mainly in the hands of the workers.

GEORGE W. TAYLOR, *Scientific Management.* An exposition of the modern type of industrial organization.

WILLIAM MORRIS, *Dream of John Ball.* Notice the emphasis on the art of the past.

PRINCE KROPOTKIN, *Fields, Factories, and Workshops.* A suggestion for rendering industry more " human ".

GALSWORTHY, *The Forsyte Saga.* A study of people who all have the possessive tendencies very strongly developed.

For types of æsthetic criticism see :

ROGER FRY, *Art and Design.* Deals with modern art.

VERNON LEE, *The Beautiful.* Principles of æsthetics.

LASCELLES ABERCROMBIE, *The Theory of Poetry.*

RICHARDS, *Principles of Literary Criticism.*

These last four books taken together give a very fair idea of the confusion of the subject and the contradictory opinions held about it.

CHAPTER VIII

THE EMOTIONS

" That's likewise part of my intelligence."

WHEN we were discussing instincts, we distinguished in them three main aspects—cognition, emotion or affect, and conation—and we pointed out that emotion generally intervened between the apprehension of a situation and the action which followed. Emotion was thus shown to be the immediate psychological precursor of action. It was also shown that the emotions were the most constant parts of an instinct. There might be very great variations in the cognitive and conative aspects of an instinct, we might fear many different things and we might show our fear in various ways, but the emotion, the feeling of fear, remained practically unaffected. Coleridge's description of intense fear would fit hundreds of different situations which give rise to the same feeling :

> Fear at my heart, as at a cup,
> My life-blood seemed to sip.[1]

The facts that emotion is the precursor of action and that emotion is nearly the same in a variety of situations make emotions a very important element in the conduct of individuals and of society. For if one can influence people's emotions, one can also probably initiate actions which can be directed to the desired ends. The process of " playing on a person's feelings ", is well known and frequently used, in school, in the family, in the police court, in church, at elections. In fact, on every occasion where one person wishes

[1] " Ancient Mariner."

to influence another's actions, he almost inevitably seeks first to raise the appropriate emotions.

Emotions seem to influence actions in several ways. In most cases, the stronger the emotion the greater the activity to which it will give rise. There are many stories told of the effects of strong emotion on action. William James records the case of an athlete, who, when a boy, was chased by a bull, and in his fright cleared a wall that he was never able to jump again till he reached his full strength. We ourselves know the energy that any strong emotion such as anger will give us, and common speech testifies to the same fact by such sayings as " fear lent him wings ".

The fact that actions follow emotions is equally clear when we consider the matter from the point of view of the action. In many people, nothing so much intensifies emotion as an inhibition of the appropriate action. It has often been maintained, though without much definite evidence in support of the theory, that, if a man runs away at the first hint of danger, he experiences little or no fear. It is certain that he experiences much less than if he tries to fly and finds his way blocked. In children's games of " prisoners and jailers " the captive, though often rather roughly handled, generally is not frightened ; but if his hands are tied, so that he feels himself helpless and unable to express himself by fight or flight, he may experience for a moment the horrors of extreme terror. In persons of an energetic and determined character each check in a course of action only serves to increase desire for the end, and so to increase the anger which is felt at being thwarted. Thus the action becomes more vigorous. We can experience something of this sort ourselves fairly frequently. We desire, faintly, to read a certain book. The library copy is lost—our desire increases. We consult a local bookseller, and he declares that it is out of print. We write to London and it has not been heard of. When finally an Oxford tradesman volunteers to supply it at a price much above what we expected, our desire is now so keen that we pay gladly, and hold the book one of our most treasured possessions, even though we never, in the end, read it.

The same kind of thing happens with children. If a child desires a certain thing, for example, an apple in his neighbour's garden, and he is prevented from getting it by a high wall, by his parents' repeated warnings of punishment to follow if he steals it, by the annoying vigilance of his neighbour's dog, and the espionage of his neighbour's son, he will probably so burn with increasing desire to get that apple that he will risk all to have it, though apples in plenty are to be had in his own kitchen.

This persistency of effort is a not infrequent theme for novelists, especially those who depict the strong, ruthless countryman with his heart set on his neighbour's plough-land. So, too, in melodrama, the terrors of a delayed and thwarted vengeance are a fairly common theme. See how Shylock's hate grows with every set-back to his scheme for vengeance !

It is, however, necessary to draw a distinction between different types of emotion. Some are of their nature active and prompt to action ; others arise in circumstances where no action is possible, and thus are depressing rather than exciting. As an example of a depressing emotion we may take great grief. We are bowed down with it, and because there is nothing to do, we are inert. If we do act it is the restless fluttering of a bird against his cage.

These two groups of emotions have radically different origins. The emotions previously described arise in the normal functioning of an instinct ; the depressing emotions afflict us when all normal outlets are checked and the instinct is utterly baulked of expression. Thus, so long as a child yet lives, a mother will lavish every tenderness and care upon it. When the child is dead, that outlet to the maternal instinct is closed ; a weight of dead sadness may now overwhelm her.

On the principle that the activity of a living organism is essentially teleological, it is natural to imagine that emotion serves some useful purpose in the life economy of the creature ; and our own experience supports this view. Emotion has two aspects, a mental and a physical, and it is in the latter aspect that the usefulness of the emotion can best be seen. Any strong emotion is accompanied by definite physical changes. In fear, or anger, we are con-scious of an increased rate of the heart-beat and of a difference in respiration. Other changes occur which are beyond our observation, but which likewise serve the purpose of making the body a more efficient machine for such violent action as is likely to be called for in flight or combat.[1] These violent emotions are naturally exhausting ; others, whose aim is rather to prompt a continuance of the present position, have a different effect. The tranquil pleasure of being with those we love leads to no violent changes, only to a general sense of well-being, and this, in turn, may have visible effects in better physical health and greater intellectual productivity.

In violent emotions, the physical aspects are so emphatically felt and seen that it has been claimed, by William James, among others, that an emotion consists entirely of the physical changes which we loosely say " accompany " it. It is hard for us to imagine such an emotion as terror without associating with it the sickening physical feeling that we know so well from nightmares ; but it is equally hard to believe that love is nothing but an alteration in the pulse and the respiration, combined with changes in certain other organs. Moreover, physiology has shown that the bodily changes accompanying such diverse emotions as fear and anger are practically the same ; so that if the whole emotions *were* the physical changes, fear and anger should be the same experience, which they are not. It is more satisfactory to regard the emotions as truly mental, and see in the bodily changes adaptations made to meet the needs of the creature in a specific set of circumstances.

A similar relation holds between the expression of the emotion in facial or other movements. It is useful to express our emotions by gesture or cry because by so doing we call the attention of others to ourselves or indicate what we are going to do. Two angry dogs, advancing towards each other, legs stiff, backs bristling, lips drawn back, show clearly that one or other must give way if he wants to avoid a fight. On the other hand, a puppy grovelling before a larger dog well expresses his pacific and humble intentions, and saves himself a beating by his submissive behaviour.

---

[1] Cannon, *Bodily Changes in Fear, Hunger, Pain and Rage.* This book is interesting for its matter and also as showing the *methods* of physiological research.

A baby calls attention to its needs or fears by a cry, and the adult indicates his feelings of pleasure or displeasure by a smile, a shrug, or other such gesture. These modes of expression are very widely spread and almost identical among men of different races and civilization. It seems probable that during man's development certain modes of expression have become " natural " to mankind. If each man had his own way of expressing anger or fear, the use of the expression as a means of communicating his state of feeling would be gone. It is the universality of the expression which makes it comprehensible and determines its utility.

Darwin in his book, *The Expression of the Emotions,* indicates three principles which he thinks determine this expression : (*a*) Some expressions are definitely useful in the activity ensuing on the emotion. Thus, when a dog in anger draws back his lips, his teeth are bared ready for the fray. When an angry or frightened cat fluffs her fur out, she makes herself look large, and is more terrible to her enemy. (*b*) Other gestures are not useful, but are the opposite of others that are, and are thus come to express an opposite emotion. Thus the fawning movements of a friendly dog are the opposite to the stiff advance of an angry one and express an opposite emotion. (*c*) Some movements seem due simply to an overflow of nervous energy and serve no purpose, *as far as we know*, e.g., the tail-switching of an angry cat.

In man, the apparent bodily expression of the emotions is largely facial or is confined to some few movements of the hands. Among certain races, as the Red Indians, or the Chinese, it is a matter of social honour to repress as far as possible any indication of emotion. This code has given rise to an elaboration of manners which cover up all the feelings of the parties concerned. Thus, in polite circles of Chinese society, if you are angry with your servant and wish to dismiss him, you tell your friend, who tells the servant that it cuts you to the heart to have to do without his, the servant's, excellent services, but owing to economic difficulties you must restrict your expenses and you will have to do with fewer servants. You can safely leave it at that, for the servant, if properly brought up, will then tell *his* friend, who will carry the message to you, that he, the servant, is desolated at the prospect, but really he finds it necessary for his health to go some fifty miles away to stay with some friends of his, and although he knows he will never be as happy again, yet he finds himself compelled for his own interest to leave your service. You receive this message with grave fortitude, the servant departs, and good manners, although they somewhat elongate, render the whole transaction dignified in the extreme, and all true expression of feeling is hidden.[1]

Among well-bred Englishmen the expression of many of the emotions is restrained. It is not good form to show your annoyance when your host's muddy dog leaps against your clean suit ; and when you are in terror of your friends reckless motor-driving, you hold tight and endeavour to say nothing. For this reason, the faces of those who are not bound by " good form " are much more interesting to look at than the faces of the rich or aristocratic. Wordsworth preferred to write of " humble and rustic life " because the peasants, he found, expressed their feelings so much more readily and truly than more sophisticated people.

If we control the outward expression of the emotion we do not necessarily control the emotion itself—although there is a widely-held theory that this is so. The lady who never told her love, but " sat like patience on a monument, smiling at grief ", found that the emotion lived, and " concealment, like a worm i' the bud, fed on her damask cheek ". The evidence on this whole question is conflicting, but as the control of emotion is a matter of great importance to each individual, we must discuss it at some length, both here and later in the book.

With little children the expression and the emotion seem more closely linked than with adults. Therefore, if one can control the expression of a child's emotions one can also control the emotion. The child has less self-control than the adult, and a very slight emotion will produce prominent symptoms. If his attention can be diverted, the emotion and its expression will both cease ; whereas if the expression is allowed to continue it will hold the child's attention and tend to prolong the emotion. If a little child falls

[1] Cf. for similar instances *The Wallet of Kai-Lung*, by Bramah.

down and begins to cry, he is told to be a brave boy and stop crying, that he is not really hurt, and will he look at the pretty horse over there. In a similar way a child in a fit of temper is reproved for smacking her sister, told to behave nicely to her, kiss and be friends, and to go and play with a new doll. The new action which is suggested draws her attention from the expression of the temper, which is thus controlled.

Even in adults some emotions can best be overcome by controlling the expression. Those who wake in the night stiff with terror know that the best way to fight the feeling is to do something active to break the spell of immobility. If one moves about, switches on the light, rustles the bed-clothes and takes deep breaths, the feeling passes. The emotion has been controlled in this case by overcoming the expressions of it.

On the other hand, some emotions seem to increase if they are denied expression or if the natural action consequent on them is prevented. If we receive an insult from a person to whom we cannot express our indignation, our anger may burn for months, and then finally burst out in a fury of passion. So did Othello's anger against Desdemona grow by concealment.

As was said before, emotion, because of its close connection with action, is important not only to the individual, but also to society. If action of a certain type is required, the easiest method of obtaining it is to stir the appropriate emotion and direct the action consequent on it to the right ends. Society, therefore, has made a considerable study of the means of arousing emotion, and makes use of them on a large variety of occasions.

When we wish to stir up emotion, the best subject on which to practise is a crowd, which is more easily stirred than a single individual. This is probably due partly to crowd sympathy ; partly to the removal of the habitual check on individual conduct which arises from a considera-tion of how our actions would appear to others. If a crowd all act together this social check is removed. In conse-quence the first act of an agitator is generally to call a meeting. When his audience is assembled various means of influencing it may be employed. The speaker may adopt the plainest method of arousing emotion and describe events or scenes which, if actually experienced, would call out the emotion. Descriptions of horror, sword and flame, famine and plunder, fire and brimstone, have formed part of the emotional speaker's stock in trade since the birth of oratory. They are as effective to-day as they were when Cicero thundered out his denunciation of Catiline, and employed his " whole paint box " of horrors.

Usually other resources are employed, which, although the psychological mechanism of them is obscure, have, doubtless, a direct effect on the emotions.

Music, rhythm, poetry—all stimulate the emotions directly. The effect is probably strongest when all three are combined, and many songs, such as the *Marseillaise*, have had an important effect in history.

> One man with a dream, at pleasure,
> Shall go forth and conquer a crown ;
> And three with a new song's measure
> Can trample a Kingdom down.[1]

Even bare rhythm can have an extraordinary effect The music of a tom-tom, or the strange gong, cymbal and trumpet bands of Tibet, can be extremely moving ; and a large part of the emotional effect of poetry depends on the movement of the verse.

Colours and their combinations have definite emotional effects, and these, in spite of certain individual differences, are fairly constant. One of the best means of studying this question is by a comparison of the posters advertising different types of plays or commodities. A combination of orange and black is more suited to melodrama than to *As You Like It*. There is a noticeable taste among the makers of beverages for a certain blue which is stimulating without being disturbing. The effects of colour are heightened by its combination with line, which also has an emotional quality of its own. No artist has used this combination more skilfully than Blake, and much of the power of his drawings depends on the vague emotional effect produced by his use of line. In advertisements the use is cruder, but the principle is the same.

[1] O'Shaughnessy, *We are the Music Makers.*

Another method of emotional stimulation is the use of lights of different colour and intensity. Arnold Bennett in his autobiography speaks regretfully of the pleasures of " liaisons under pink lampshades ", which he never experienced, and for many people the idea of a flirtation implies suitably shaded and coloured lights. The theatre makes abundant use of this emotional stimulation—cold blue light for the deed of horror, crimson for the police court scene, purple moonlight for lovers' passions ; and, though for a totally different purpose, so does religion.

Certain arts or organizations regularly employ all, or most, of these stimulants to emotion. A political meeting will be gay with flags, loud with party songs, and excited by the eloquence of the speaker. Opera gives us music, light, colour, and the imitation of action. The gorgeous trappings of *Chu Chin Chow* aroused emotions strong enough to overcome for the time being the fears of war. That is why *Chu Chin Chow* succeeded in war-time, and its imitators fail during peace, when we have less need of such stimulation. In a ritualistic church slow-moving, gorgeously apparelled priests focus our attention on the service of God, and all the accessories stir us to devotion :

> The high embowe'd roof,
> With antique pillars massy proof,
> And storied windows richly dight,
> Casting a dim religious light.
> There let the pealing organ blow,
> To the full-voiced quire below,
> In service high, and anthems clear,
> As may with sweetness, through mine ear,
> Dissolve me into ecstasies,
> And bring all Heaven before mine eyes.

The aim of this socially-aroused emotion is generally action. A political meeting is expected to bear fruit at the polls, and religion should affect life. The most remarkable example of the large scale attempt to arouse emotion for a definite purpose occurred in 1914 and 1915 when the government was trying to raise recruits for the army. Speeches were made, patriotic songs published, posters covered the walls, the church lent its authority, old maids their officiousness. Detestation of Germany, admiration for our allies, wrath and fear for ourselves were stirred by all means possible, and the practical result, which the authorities hoped would follow all this emotion, was enlistment.

Not all emotion, however, is stimulated with a practical aim in view. Many emotions are, in themselves, pleasant, and we stimulate them for their own sakes. Such, for example, is the emotion aroused by a dance. Such again are the experiences that we get from listening to good music, or any form of art. In religion there is a prostration before the infinite which is wonderfully satisfying to some natures.

There are certain emotions which, if present in a strong degree, would be painful, but which, if experienced in a milder form, are pleasant, and which are therefore sought for their own sake. The " thrills " of a scenic railway or the films stir our fear slightly, the misfortunes of the hero or heroine of tragedy may move us to tears, yet we come home saying that it was a " beautiful play ". The cause of the pleasure which we derive from tragedy has long been a matter of speculation. Aristotle in the *Poetics* said that witnessing a tragedy effected a " purgation of the feelings of pity and terror ", and, therefore, left us freer of these emotions in our daily life. This theory accounts for the relief we experience *after* an emotional outburst, but not for our satisfaction at the time. Freud has suggested that we triumph in the hero's fall because we unconsciously look upon him as a rival. This also is untrue, because in a good tragedy the tendency is to identify ourselves to a large extent with the hero. The explanation is perhaps far simpler than any of these. All the powers that man possesses require use, and if they are not exercised they cause discomfort. This is most obvious in the case of muscles, and hygiene invariably prescribes physical exercise. It is also fairly obvious with mental powers—to be deprived of mental exercise for more than a few days is to many people as trying as to be deprived of physical. In the same way, when our lives follow a smooth and easy course, we enjoy emotional stimulation even of a slightly painful kind.[1]

[1] Those of us who lead fairly safe, comfortable lives, find a strange comfort in the poems of A. E. Housman. On the other hand, A. A. Milne, in the trenches during the Great War, wrote comedies.

In certain people a liking for emotions for their own sake becomes a vice ; in those people, that is, for whom emotion becomes disconnected from action, and therefore loses its primary biological use. Such people are generally known as sentimentalists. They become wrapped up in their own feelings and live for them. They are normally the product of a state of society in which individual effort is not greatly called for. They are more common among the classes who do not have to work for their living than among those who do. The rich, of course, lead easier lives and are more secure, and therefore circumstances do not insist on action as the needs of the poor man do.

Duke Orsino in *Twelfth Night* is a sentimentalist in love. He enjoys all the thrill of the emotion, experienced with its due accompaniments of music and " beds of flowers ", but not until it is too late does he attempt by his own efforts to woo Olivia. Jaques in *As You Like It* is a type of the melancholy sentimentalist enjoying his woe as a luxury. Other examples are to be found in the hypochondriacs who " enjoy " bad health.

Some nations have satisfied this sentimental craving for emotion in the most brutal ways. The Minoan lords of Crete employed boy and girl athletes for bull fights, which, to judge by the story of Theseus, were extremely dangerous. The Spaniards of to-day have bull fights, but the later Roman Republic and Early Empire satisfied these tastes to an extent unparalled in European history. Vast numbers of animals were hunted and slaughtered in the arena, while gladiatorial fights were a commonplace, and Christians and criminals were put to more diverting deaths.

Of course, the taste for horrors is not a monopoly of any class, and coarser imaginations need more violent stimuli. As long as hanging was public, a crowd would gather to watch the death agony ; now the thrill has to be enjoyed in the more remote form of a newspaper report, but the law courts are still crowded by folk who gloat upon the thrilling details and sensational suffering of a murderer or a divorced woman

Emotion has very pronounced effects on the intellectual processes. In the first place, strong emotion will so dominate our minds that we are incapable, during the sway of emotion, of normal reasoning or thought. For thought or reasoning we need to bring into connexion various ideas ; in strong emotion we are incapable of attending to more than the one. In consequence it is vain to reason with a person in anger. He may listen to argument when the fit is over ; at the moment, the prudent course is to bow before the storm. A milder degree of emotion will not confine us to a single idea, but to a single type of ideas. When we feel thoroughly depressed we cannot see a joke, and to read *Punch* at such a time is sheer waste. William James records how the misery due to sea-sickness entirely changed his view of *The Three Musketeers*. If, on the other hand, we are feeling gay, our friends' misfortunes are for the time forgotten. Young lovers feel that all the earth shares their happiness.

The connective force of congruent emotions does much to explain the formation of similes in a poet's mind. Two objects in experience arouse the same or similar emotion, and being thus connected, the one is used to explain or illustrate the other. A very simple case is such a simile as

> My love is like a red, red rose
> That's newly sprung in June
> My love is like a melody
> That's sweetly played in tune.

Far more complicated are similes like those in Shelley's *Ode to the West Wind* :

> O wild west wind, thou breath of Autumn's being,
> Thou, from whose unseen presence the leaves dead
> Are driven, like ghosts from an enchanter fleeing,
> Yellow and black, and pale and hectic red
> Pestilence-stricken multitudes.

It is easy to see how the fair beauty of a lady and her gracious presence suggest roses and melodies, but it is necessary to know something of Shelley's life, his early experiments in magic, and his horror of war and the ravages of poverty, before we can understand how those similes came to suggest themselves to him.

The poet depends on the association of emotion with

certain images to create "atmosphere". Coleridge is a past master of this art:

> The water, like a witch's oils,
> Burnt green, and blue, and white.

> Her skin was white as leprosy.

> A savage place,
> As holy and enchanted,
> As e'er beneath a waning moon was haunted
> By woman wailing for her demon lover.

The force of these similes depends on the fact that they produce the desired emotions in nearly every reader.

Emotion has a strong effect on memory, but this effect is sometimes contradictory. If an event is accompanied by a strong emotional tone, it is very likely to persist in memory. In some cases this event may continually recur to memory and become an obsession. This is well known. On the other hand, we sometimes find that an event, which was accompanied at its occurrence by a strong unpleasant emotion, has been forgotten by the sufferer. This forgetfulness is often complete, and it may only be possible to recover the memory by the use of some special device. Such lost memories are the special concern of psychoanalysis and will be spoken of later. Short, however, of such complete forgetfulness, unpleasant emotion may work against a memory. The schoolboy who was taught Latin with the rod made far less progress, considering the time that was devoted to the subject, than the modern boy taught by milder methods. The greater pleasantness of the feeling tone accompanying learning in modern times has much to do with the change, although improvements in other directions are not without their salutary influence.

FOR DISCUSSION

1.—Study on a cinema film the bodily expressions of various emotions in man, and see how far Darwin's principles can be applied to them.
2.—What means of raising corporate emotion can we use in schools, and for what purposes should they be used?
3.—What are the chief differences between the account of emotion given in W. James's *Text Book* and McDougall's *Social Psychology*? Give your opinion about the points at issue.

THE EMOTIONS

4.—Study the emotions displayed by, e.g., a cat or dog, and compare them with those of man as regards their origin, number, etc.

5.—What do you think of the work of such writers of animal stories as Thompson Seton in regard to their portrayal of animal character.

6.—Discuss the effect of any strong widely-spread emotion on the life of a nation, e.g., *fear* (cf. Tacitus, histories of French Revolution, Czarist Russia) or *positive self feeling* (cf. Victorian England, Germany before the Great War).

7.—Discuss the emotional value to the nation of (*a*) Hitler's persecution of the Jews or (*b*) Mussolini's conquest of Abyssinia.

BOOKS

MacCunn, *The Making of Character*. Read this selectively in connection with this and later chapters. It is a useful exposition of the traditional view which is rapidly going out of fashion.

Yeats, *The King's Threshold*. A short play on the right of the poet to a place in the councils of the nation.

Baudouin, *Studies in Psycho-Analysis*, Pt. ii, Ch. ii. This shows the connection between the images of poetry and dreams, and the affective origin of both.

Tacitus, *Annals*, esp. Bk. xiv., Ch. 41 to end, and Bk. xv., Nero's reign of terror. Note the different effect on different characters. cf. also books on Russia given at end of Ch. iv.

CHAPTER IX

SENTIMENTS

" I love my love with an A, because she is amiable."

THEORETICALLY any object might, according to circumstances, arouse any emotion ; actually we find that this is not so. Certain objects or persons or ideals become the centre of a definitely organized group of emotions, and such a group is called a sentiment.

If we have a sentiment for a thing, we tend to feel more strongly for it than for other objects of the same kind for which we have no sentiment. Thus, a person develops a sentiment for a room in which he has played, for the tree at which trysts have been kept, or for his school ; and his emotional reaction to these particular things is quite different from his feelings regarding rooms, trees and schools in general. We feel a thrill of pleasure at returning to old haunts, or when good news comes of our school. "Forty years on, when afar and asunder ", memories of the "great days in the distance enchanted " can still awaken a very real throb of pleasure. Conversely our anger, our fear, or sympathy, is most quickly stirred if the objects of our sentiments are assailed or in danger.

Often, indeed, we remain almost ignorant of the fact that we possess a sentiment for a thing until that thing is attacked ; and then. we are surprised at the passion and feeling we experience, and say, " I had no idea I cared so much."

Sentiments seem to grow deeper, and to change in character with experience. They are the product of emotional experiences had in connection with a thing, and every particular experience adds a little to the development of the particular sentiment.

Thus my mother bought me a doll which at first sight won my heart, with its light-blue eyes and " real " hair and attractive green frock. Day after day, the undressing and dressing of the doll was a delightful experience, until the time came when I was too old to take such pleasure in public. Then came the secret communes with the faded tattered object, beautiful and beloved to me, and to this day, in my drawer, as surely in the drawers of thousands of other grown women, are the remains of this loved object—kept, as we say, for " sentimental reasons ". The experiences have left a tendency to feel for the object, quite out of proportion to the present actual value of the object itself.

Many treasures of this kind are not the actual thing which gave pleasure in the first place, but something connected with it—a ring, a book, a letter from a beloved person. Popular drawing-room ballads are full of references to such examples :

> I love it, I love it, and who shall dare
> To chide me for loving that old arm chair :
> I treasured it long as a sainted prize,

and the reason for this ill-expressed but widely shared experience, is the fact that " a mother sat there—and a sacred thing is that old arm chair ". The sentiment has been transferred. So do symbols, monuments, cenotaphs, tombstones and relics become hallowed.

A sentiment normally develops to include not only an object or person connected with the original experience, but also an abstract ideal or idea. Such sentiments are of the highest importance in the moral life. Virtue may be knowledge, but we do not act virtuously unless our emotions drive us to action. Few sins are committed through *ignorance* of what is right and wrong, they are due rather to indifference about it. But if we have a tendency to feel strongly, to care greatly for certain ideals, we shall be more likely to act in accordance with them than we should be if we merely knew of them.

The growth of such sentiments can be seen on every

hand. A child loves his father, and many are the jolly experiences they have together. These pleasurable experiences are due partly to instinctive satisfaction in being with his parent, partly to admiration of the father's prowess and power to amuse. A sentiment is formed for the father. The father cares for animals. The child sees this, and, tending to identify himself with his father, sympathizes with the feeling. In after years he will be kind to animals " for his father's sake ", and so be led, maybe, to a true and first-hand feeling for the ideal on its own merits.

The growth of Wordsworth's attitude to Nature, described in *The Prelude*, is an excellent example of how a sentiment grows from the instinctive, concrete, particular stage to the philosophic, abstract and universal ideal. The peaks and lakes of his native Cumberland were the objects of many experiences of love and of fear. Unthinking, and devoid of " any interest not borrowed from the eye ", he bounded like a roe amongst the hills. When he returned home from Cambridge as a young man, he realized how deep his feeling for the mountains, and clouds, and rivers, and for the peasants had grown. The sentiment, that is, became conscious and more inclusive. It was the cause of the mystic, passionate experiences he described in his poem :

> . . . that serene and blessed mood,
> In which the affections gently lead us on—
> Until, the breath of this corporeal frame
> And even the motion of our human blood
> Almost suspended, we are laid asleep
> In body, and become a living soul :
> And see into the life of things.[1]

From this stage he began to feel, not only for the concrete individual forms of Nature, but for a Being, a Spirit,

> Whose dwelling is the light of setting suns,
> And the round ocean and the living air,
> And the blue sky, and in the mind of man.[1]

Hence developed his philosophy of Nature and of Life, for which he cared with increasing fervour ; for this senti-

[1] *Tintern Abbey.*

ment was the growth of a life-time, enriched with countless emotional experiences, and with its roots in the unreflective pleasure of youth.

A kind of negative sentiment can be formed by experiences which savour of the unpleasant ; such sentiments we should call antipathies. " I never see that place without shuddering ; it is where I spent the most unhappy weeks of my life " Many antipathies towards noble ideals have been formed by unpleasant experiences endured in connection with them. Such were the agonies of the Presbyterian Sabbath, or the dreary catechising lessons of the last century.

Sentiments, therefore, play an extremely important part in our lives ; they are the units of mental, emotional organization, and remain comparatively stable. Therefore, from an educational point of view, sentiments are very important. If we can train a person's emotional reactions, we also largely determine his action ; if we can bring it about that the emotions experienced are those that we desire, we have a good prospect of securing suitable action. It must, then, be an important part of education to see that the sentiments formed by a child are in accordance with the needs of society.

Sentiments formed for abstract objects have generally been helped by training and do not spring up without instruction.

There are two factors in the formation of a sentiment— an intellectual comprehension of the object of the sentiment, and the organization of emotion round that object. In sentiments formed for concrete objects the former factor is so simple as to cause no trouble. If we learn to love our home or our parents, we have no difficulty in comprehending the object of our affection, but if we are to love justice we must know what is just, what unjust ; and this is not always easy. For this reason a large part of the teaching directed to forming sentiments for moral ideals is occupied in pointing out what is right or wrong, honest or dishonest, tidy or untidy. Concurrently with this intellectual teaching, the teacher tries to attach pleasurable emotions to that particular class of actions which are the outcome of the desired ideal, and painful ones to the opposite. Unkind actions may be blamed, kind ones praised, lies may be punished, untidy work returned, or tidy exercises pinned up on the wall for general admiration. In stories, good deeds may receive their reward and the wicked man become like chaff. Thus the teacher hopes to create a sentiment for the kind boy, the tidy child, the brave hero, and ultimately for kindness, tidiness and bravery.

A consideration of the formation of one particular sentiment will show the way in which educationalists try to influence their pupils. In many schools an attempt is made to teach patriotism and a devotion to the British Empire. We can distinguish various elements in this teaching.

(a) *The Intellectual Element.*—(1) This is generally given in geography lessons, which tell of the size and character of the Empire. In its crudest form it is closely connected with a map of the world with the Dominions marked in red ; in its best form it attempts to give a real understanding of, and sympathy with the lives of distant peoples.

(2) Besides knowing what they are to love, children need to be shown the way in which their love should be expressed. They are, therefore, taught—largely in history —the deeds of eminent patriots. Too often in the past, militarist tradition has confined the list of heroes to warriors, but to-day explorers, missionaries, nurses, philanthropists, doctors, all have their place, and children are given a wide range of heroes to venerate and models to imitate.

(b) *The Emotional Element.*—(1) Lessons which hold up the lives of great men to admiration, necessarily stir emotion, and it might be good to leave the matter there, rather than employ the more sensational methods which may provoke disgust and disillusionment in the fastidious. With older school children Empire Day celebrations, with their inevitable suggestion of Jingoism and " lesser breeds without the law ", frequently have an effect quite contrary to that intended by the organizers, but with younger and less critical children there is less danger.

(2) Methods of deliberately evoking emotion include school services, hymns, poems, bands and flags. The

emotion aroused by these means could be directed to almost any aim, as such excitants of emotion are employed indiscriminately in countless causes, but in school the emotion is given a specific turn and directed to the intellectual ideas of patriotism which have previously been formed. If the scheme is successful, the sentiment formed should lend enough force to these ideas to make them issue in action of a serviceable kind.

There is the same ætiology for other sentiments, though the exact methods used differ according to the sentiment which it is desired to form. Thus the celebrations on Armistice Day differ from those of Empire Day, because in one it is the sacrifices of patriotism which are emphasized, and in the other the pride of rule.

Among the sentiments formed in school, love of tidiness and cleanliness take an important place. Too often such virtues are spoken of as *habits*, and then their real nature is obscured. A habit operates only within a limited sphere under circumstances which have become stereotyped, and a change in the circumstances is very likely to break the habit. A sentiment is more adaptable and more reliable.[1] A child may form a habit of doing sums tidily, but be extremely untidy at home or in other work ; a real love of, or sentiment for tidiness will show itself in all branches of life. In fact, the aim of a teacher in regard to morals should be to build up sentiments of love for the virtues, since by this means, far more than by hatred of the vices, can a stable and lovable character be formed.

The moral character of a man depends mainly on the sentiments he has formed, since these provide him with his normal reactions to situations, and also with an emotional force sufficient to make him act according to his ideals. The whole question of character is discussed later.

The inhabitants of any one country have a large mass of common sentiments which form the general moral code of the race, but there are considerable differences from country to country, age to age, or even among different social ranks in the same society. Many people who have access to books incorporate in their character sentiments of

[1] McDougall, *Outline of Psychology*, Ch. xvii.

an age or country other than their own, since many sentiments which are held valuable under one set of circumstances
are disregarded in another. To take an instance—it is
illegal in England to commit suicide, and an unsuccessful
attempt may be punished by imprisonment. Moreover,
most people think that suicide is a moral crime and shrink
from the idea of it. In other countries or ages suicide has
been, not a crime, but a virtue.[1] In Imperial Rome it was
an everyday occurrence, and there were fashions in death
as in clothes.[2] To-day, in times of political disturbance,
suicide by hunger-striking may make a man a martyr.
So, too, with homicide, which is a crime in peace, a virtue
in war ; or with spying, a deed of patriotism if done by a
fellow countryman, a base act on the part of enemy subjects. Duelling is dead in England, and flickers on the
Continent, yet two hundred years ago a gentleman was
obliged to fight when suitably challenged.

If we are to bring about a change in the morals of a nation,
we must set ourselves to build up the sentiments most
influential in effecting the conduct we desire. These
must first be sought out and the means of forming them
studied. The schools have a great influence in this respect, and the effect of their teaching can be seen comparatively rapidly. Twenty years ago one could often see
boys in the street tormenting a cat or some other animal ;
the schools have started Nature Study and encouraged
children to be interested in and kind to animals ; now it is
very rare to see an act of cruelty. If such are done, they
are performed in secrecy and shame.

To-day in many schools a conscious attempt is being
made to form a sentiment for the League of Nations by
teaching world history, world geography, and by interesting children in the problems of other lands. Other sentiments which receive attention are a love of beauty and
cleanliness ; and an interest in the open air and physical
exercise.

[1] Cf. story of Lucretia or Cato the Younger.
[2] Tacitus, op cit.

SENTIMENTS

FOR DISCUSSION

1.—What do you think are the most important sentiments, from the point of view of the good of society, that can be developed in school ? What means would you adopt to inculcate them ?
2.—Why do we seek to win the children's love for their school ?
3.—Distinguish carefully between sentiment and sentimentality. How would you deal with a child of fifteen who you thought was becoming a sentimentalist ?
4.—Why do promoters of popular plays, tales and cinema films find it pays to make much use of " sob stuff " ?
5.—What methods does the Boy Scouts Organization adopt to inculcate a sentiment for the ideal of competent service and of good health ?
6.—What objects of beauty are within the reach of children in your district ? In what way would you try to surround them with beauty as Plato suggests in the *Republic* ?
7.—Mention a number of stories that you would use to inculcate virtues in a child, and say what points in them you would stress, and what effect you hope they would have. Do you remember any stories that had a strong effect on you ?

BOOKS

MacCunn, *Making of Character.* Pt. ii., Ch. ix., x., xi., and Pt. iii.
Graham Wallas, *Human Nature in Politics*, Ch. ii. The formation of sentiments in politics or commerce.
Plato, *Republic.* End of Bk. ii. and beginning of Bk. iii. A discussion of the type of story to be used for the formation of character. The myth of Er at the end of Bk. x. is an example of the type of story he would think suitable.
Shakespeare, *Richard II.* An excellent picture of a sentimentalist.
Wordsworth, *The Prelude. Tintern Abbey.*

CHAPTER X

THE SELF-REGARDING SENTIMENT AND THE WILL

" Swear by thy gracious self."

WE deliberately left one of the most important sentiments out of consideration in the last chapter, because it is so closely connected with the main subject of the present one. The more developed forms of will depend on the self-regarding sentiment, and this sentiment is partly dependent on that consciousness of personal effort which may be called will.

A child early distinguishes himself from his surroundings. He learns what he can feel and do, and he learns the distinction between himself and other persons, and between living people and inanimate things. There follows a stage in which a child is conscious of himself as a living being, but not conscious of himself as an object of his own thought. This last stage can only come through experience of the action of other human beings. It is not natural to turn back and consider oneself—to say : " I want to take my sister's doll, but I should do wrong if I did that." This power of reflection and self-criticism is the result of social interaction. A child, who is conscious of himself as a spring of energy, is treated by others as an object to be judged, praised, or reproved. He learns by degrees to think of himself under two aspects —as a thinking being, and also as an object of thought. Hence arise, at a later stage, all the philosophical difficulties of the " ego ", and problems of the identity of that " self " which lies behind the particular events of everyday life, and which passes judgment on its own acts.

From this double aspect also arises the self-regarding sentiment. Each person forms the idea of himself as an object, and round this object emotions gather as round any other. The two main emotions involved are those noticed in the description of the herd instinct as arising in connection with leadership and following, or with the praise or blame of others. But all the other emotions can be involved—for the " self " feels all the emotions, and can also make these emotions the object of its thought. This is what many people habitually do, and thus their mental state is almost always a complex one.

For example, they are angry and know that they are; that is, they experience the emotion and are conscious of it, but they also consider that the causes of the anger are inadequate, and that they are wrong to experience so much feeling on so slight a provocation. Thus they make their anger the object of critical thought. All this is not felt successively but simultaneously and blended into one state of feeling.

On the other hand, there are many people who experience this dual attitude seldom. They remain in the childish state of absorption in the emotion of the moment. They are happy or sad, excited or depressed, and they act simply and directly according to their emotion. Only occasionally is a criticism of their behaviour forced on them. There are some people who will not accept this criticism unless it is very sharp ; others are more sensitive, but the criticism still has to come from without, and is not the internal running commentary on their actions that it is with others. There is little doubt that the unself-critical are on the whole the happier ; the critical are probably easier to live with.

Most people, whatever their type, form a definite idea of themselves as being of such-and-such a character, and as possessing such-and-such qualities and capabilities. This idea is partly forced on us by the way we are treated, and partly is formed by our own thought. A pretty child soon realizes its beauty by the treatment it receives from others. A clever child is praised and finds itself top of the form. The charming are greeted with smiles, the unattractive find everyone difficult to get on with.

In addition we form some ideal of conduct and behaviour for ourselves.

We may in our thoughts liken ourselves to saints or heroes, and then, though we know our model unattainable, we strive towards it ; or we may, if we are folk of more ordinary type, form an opinion of ourselves as "no worse than our neighbours", and refrain from conduct which would outrage this conception of ourselves. A common appeal of moralists and teachers is made to this idea of self. "That is unworthy of you—you lower yourself in doing that," they say. To ourselves we say, "That is beneath me, I cannot sink to that." Thus we refer conduct to our idea of ourselves, which becomes a standard.

This fact is important in training children. To a large extent they will become what they think of themselves as being. A boy who in his thoughts regards himself as honest, hardworking and truthful, will be filled with shame when it is pointed out to him that he is not doing his best or has told a lie. A boy who has come to regard himself as a "bad lot" regards his sins rather as a confirmation of his previous opinion and hence as a source of pride. A good instance of pride in stupid acts is provided by the boy who regards himself as a "devil of a fellow", and recounts all kinds of unsavoury episodes with vaunting pride. On the other hand, the phrase, "No decent fellow does that," implies that the speaker holds himself a "decent fellow", and will therefore abstain.

This conception of ourselves is, thus, arrived at in various ways. It is due partly to our own native endowments and character ; partly to the way in which others treat us. As the flower-girl says in Shaw's *Pygmalion* :

"You see, really and truly, apart from the things that anyone can pick up (the dressing and the proper way of speaking, and so on) the difference between a lady and a flower-girl is not how she behaves, but how she is treated. . . . I know I can be a lady to you, because you always treat me as a lady and always will."

A child who is taught to believe that he is essentially good, though subject to lapses which effort may cure, has a better chance of really becoming good than one who is always being told that he is " a naughty boy " and likely " to come to a bad end ". In school, therefore, we must refrain from labelling A as a dunce, or B as untidy, or C as a nuisance. They quickly adopt this view of themselves and live up to it.

We can notice this difference of attitude in ourselves in regard to different objects. If we consider ourselves musical, to be told that we are singing out of tune is insulting ; if we are tone deaf, and the same thing happens, we smile complacently and say, " Yes, of course, *I* never *could* sing in tune." The same thing applies in other subjects. Some of us cannot write good English, do mathematics, or spell ; we are so used to being told of these faults that we have incorporated them into our idea of ourselves and make little effort to overcome them.

To bring about a reformation in character it is necessary to re-establish a person's self-respect. This fact is now widely recognized, and is part of the policy of those engaged in prison reform. A man with no self-respect offers no handle to the reformer, he has no sense of shame, and is no more abashed than Falstaff when his lies and his cowardice are proved against him.[1] The effect of this self-regarding sentiment on the higher forms of will should be clear later.

The difficulty in discussing the will lies in the different senses in which the word is used. For some writers " will " is the power of sustained voluntary activity which develops out of the fitful striving seen in children or animals. In this sense it appears as " determination ", " persistence ", " concentration of effort " ; and a man who, on his own initiative, conscientiously devotes eight hours a day to solid work, is said to be " strong-willed ". For other writers " will " is deliberate action in the line of greatest resistance, this action being prompted by a consideration of the worth of the action. Thus if we want very much to go to a dance, but know we should finish an essay, we are conscious of a struggle in our minds, and if we decide to finish the essay, we have a sense of having willed to do so. We say that a person who is able

[1] *Henry IV.*, Part I, Act ii., Sc. 4.

frequently to resist such temptations is strong-willed. It is well to take these two meanings of " will " separately.

" Will " as the power of sustained voluntary effort can be observed to grow with age and training. A little child, like a cat, shows little fixity of purpose or continuity of effort. A cat provides many illustrations of this point. Recently one of the writers was watching a cat trying to catch a field-mouse. The creature had taken cover among the stems of a tiny laurel bush, and the cat was walking round making scoops with his paw at the cowering mouse. He could not reach far enough to touch the mouse, but hoped to frighten it out into the open. Though he was clearly much interested in the mouse his attention was unstable : every now and then he stopped to look up or down the garden, and then, after an interval, resumed his hunting. A similar course of action can be seen when a cat sends a ball, with which he is playing, under a piece of furniture. He tries to get it out, but his efforts are interrupted by walks about the room, or he lies down and gets up to try again. There is a fairly persistent purpose (a cat may continue to try to get the ball for some time), but no sustained effort.

A little child is not much more developed in this direction than a cat, and is quite incapable of anything like the adult's long-continued application to a task. Much of the training given in school is directed to helping the children to acquire this power of continuous effort. The children are expected to devote their minds for comparatively long periods to certain work which is often of a not very interesting nature.

Owing to a certain confusion of thought, it is often assumed that unless the work is uninteresting it is not serving the purpose for which it is intended. It was felt that if a child was given practice in attending, he was training a general power of " will " which could be turned to all kinds of uses in life. Thus, if a boy could be made to plod through two weary hours of uninteresting long multiplication sums, he would mechanically develop a power of " will " which would enable him to apply his efforts with equal persistence to carpentry, reading or digging. It sometimes happens, of course, that a boy who does so apply himself to uninteresting tasks in school applies himself also to uninteresting drudgery out of the school; but this fact is not necessarily a result of the " exercise " given by the unpleasant task, it may result from many causes. Indeed, persistent effort is not in itself a virtue. It may be due to a lack of the imagination to suggest more profitable and interesting ways of spending one's time, or to sheer inertia, which will not trouble to change a job : when one is very tired, one often finds oneself jogging on with work, merely because one is too tired to stop. One becomes stupidly mechanical. We need not mere persistency, but persistency in pursuit of a useful aim ; and, though the idea of ourselves as hard workers is a very good thing, it is important that we should not exhaust ourselves by labour for worthless ends.

So long as will is used in the sense in which we are now using it, any continued activity is an exercise of it, and much is gained if the exercise can be made attractive, so that the child has *pleasurable* experiences of continuous activity which will aid in forming a sentiment for such conduct.

Acting, drawing, singing, handwork or games, as well as ordinary lessons train will in this sense, and perhaps games train it most of all, because here the effort of playing and attending must be continued even when physical fatigue begins to set in. Dull lessons frequently defeat their own object. The children, unable to attend to the matter in hand, develop a capacity for mind wandering and day-dreaming which is a hindrance to work in later life. The teacher has, then, no moral obligation to be dull.

When used in the sense of persistent effort, will is a direct development of the instinctive unorganized impulses ; in the other sense of deliberate action along the line of greatest resistance, it involves the acceptance by the individual of certain standards of conduct. When we hesitate between two courses of conduct and prefer one because it seems to us to be the higher, we have in mind both an evaluation of different types of conduct and also an idea of ourselves as choosing the nobler.

The evaluation of types of conduct is the result of the training we have received, and is the expression of the moral sentiments that we have formed. The idea of ourselves is due to the formation of the self-regarding sentiment which thus actually determines our will. Without this element a knowledge of right and wrong would be useless. If I am "determined to prove a villain ",[1] I shall not take the better course even if I know it ; rather my moral knowledge will *the more* surely guide me to crime. Without a formed idea of the self the weaker motive would be helpless against the urgency of more immediate desire, and though a man might praise virtue he would fail to avoid vice.

This type of will is, therefore, best cultivated by increasing the self-respect of the child and by giving him noble ideals ; it is not to be achieved by a depressingly rigid discipline nor by the imposition of irksome tasks which irritate or deaden.

Will in both senses is a good thing, yet a generation or so ago there was much talk of "breaking a child's will ", and the dangers that would follow if he were left to grow up " self-willed ".

The reason for this was that the earliest manifestations of what may be called will are the actions prompted by the different instincts, and these are frequently a-social if not anti-social. But these instincts are the fount of all energy to whatever end it may be directed, so that the proper method of dealing with them is by sublimation, not by any attempt to eradicate them. This was not always realized in the past, and more intelligence is needed for one course than the other. It used to be assumed that the education of children was an easy thing, well within the power of any "motherly woman ", and did not need any particular thought. The rod was not spared, and a tradition sprang up. Parents, having had to suffer repression in their own youth, used their paternal power in their turn to satisfy their instincts of self-assertion, and expected complete submissiveness from their children.[2] This flattered the parents' pride ; but its result

[1] Cf. *Richard III.*, Act I., Sc. I. The whole speech should be studied for its psychological insight.

[2] Cf. the state of things represented in, e.g., *Vanity Fair*, or by the " hard father " of the melodramas.

was often not to train, but to destroy the children's will, or else to drive the unfortunate child into abnormal resistance and self-assertion.

Further, children frequently refuse to do things that are good for them. They will not go to school or clean their teeth, and then, in so far as they cannot be persuaded peacefully, a certain amount of force must be employed ; but punishment is only a last resource. A child who can be brought to like school or enjoy cleanliness is far better than one who only suffers these things from fear, and would be untaught and unwashed if he dared.

Obedience may be given by one person to another for various reasons ; the best are love and respect, the worst is fear. To obey through fear is the lot of a slave, and no child should be put in that position.

A strong will, if it be directed to good aims, is one of the most valuable possessions a person can have. This " strength " of will arises from various causes. It is partly due to a natural vividness of desire which seems to vary in different people ; it is partly due, as we have seen, to the strength of the self-regarding sentiment.

Men whose " will " to achieve some great end has been indefatigable, have generally been blessed with extraordinary vividness of desire. They become so convinced of the reality of the end at which they aim that the difficulties, sneers of others, and even their own ill-health and natural incapacity are overcome. To Abraham Lincoln, the vision of a United States of America, in which there should be no slavery, was so real that all his powers could be directed unflinchingly to attaining that end. Milton's vision of himself as the author of a great poem, " so written to after times as they would not willingly let it die ", was vivid enough to outlive the twenty years' distraction of civil war. Most " iron-wills " and unflinching determinations can be thus analysed into a vivid desire for some result on the one hand, and on the other a strong sentiment for a certain ideal of oneself as the creator or achiever of the situation seen in the vision.

As the self-regarding sentiment is only built up during childhood, and as some people are born with a tendency to desire greatly, many people who have strong wills in later life are naughty children. They want things violently, and, knowing no better, seek to break down opposition to their desire by a display of anger. They scream and kick, sometimes do damage in their fury, and are best left alone till the fit is over. But with time this changes. The child learns to regard such displays of temper as useless and undignified ; if he learns self-respect, he realizes that such displays do not fit in with his ideal of himself. He discovers that it is often easier to get what one wants by smooth words than by rough, and he learns to desire a noble character for himself as much as he previously desired his neighbour's toy. The naughty child is, therefore, not to be met by punishment so much as by persuasion. His will is not to be " broken ", but trained, and nobler desires must be substituted for the anti-social tendencies of childhood. He needs also to be taught the way in which ends are achieved—by honourable policy and adroit consideration for others. If this training is successful, the naughty child, in his young manhood, studies the social arts, and wins that place by good manners which he could never have achieved by violence.

FOR DISCUSSION

1.—Distinguish carefully between " strong will " and obstinacy or " pig-headedness ".
2.—Try to give a psychological account of " conscience ", i.e., say how it appears to operate in yourself, what gives force to its promptings, whence it gets its standard of right and wrong, and how it changes.
3.—What do you mean when you speak of having " free will " ?
4.—Give an account of any methods or organizations that are used in school to allow the children to exercise their own wills in various ways.
5.—Is it possible or desirable " to harden " a child when young so that he will be more easily able to withstand the difficulties of life ?
6.—What tasks in school seem still to be mainly drudgery ? Is drudgery in any way educational ? If not, how could it be made so ?
7.—What part do and should prizes and rewards play in training children to sustain interest in prolonged routine work ?
8.—What are the peculiar dangers and difficulties that beset a person with an abnormally " strong will " ?

BOOKS

JOHN DEWEY, *Educational Essays*, Ch. ii. A discussion of interest in work versus drudgery. See also the chapter on " Attention " in this book.

McDOUGALL, *Social Psychology*. The chapters on this topic are most important.

SAMUEL BUTLER, *The Way of All Flesh*. A novel based on self-assertion from one generation to another.

WILLIAM JAMES, *Talks to Teachers*. The chapter on the will is interesting, especially when compared with M Dougall's account.

J. S. MILL, *Utilitarianism*. In one chapter there is an excellent psychological account of conscience.

CHAPTER XI

WORK AND MOTIVES FOR EFFORT

Half-a-pound of tuppenny rice
Half-a-pound of treacle . . .

THROUGHOUT the animal kingdom there is a fairly general expenditure of effort in the attempt to live. Some creatures seem to do it with much less exertion than others—the axolotl is almost unbelievably lethargic and the bee incredibly busy—but all have to do something. In man this expenditure of effort becomes very great and is often very persistent. The interesting thing from the psychological point of view is that this effort frequently goes beyond that necessary for earning a living. This is particularly the case with the Northern races. As we approach the equator the standard of effort decreases, and we get races that, by Northern standards, appear as hopelessly lethargic as the axolotl. This is in many cases due to disease. In certain countries, e.g., Ceylon, the great bulk of the population is infected with malaria and hookworm, two diseases that enormously reduce the possibility of effort. But there are other races, e.g., the Zulus, who are on the whole healthy and live in an invigorating climate, where the men, if they can, do no work and leave all the necessary cultivation to the women, while they sit in the sun and tell stories. With the Zulus this is almost certainly the legacy of their great fighting days, for, by immemorial custom, the warrior does not work on the land.

It is claimed by those who defend the custom of keeping animals in small pens in Zoological Gardens that animals are lazy and if they are provided with food ask nothing better than to sleep their time away. This is patently untrue, and the poor bored animals are a pathetic refutation of this theory. Even the well-fed domestic cat kills for pleasure, though he may not eat his kill. In man, Northern man, the necessity and liking for effort seems to be well established ; and without the opportunity for effort his life becomes aimless and dissolute. A very brief sketch of attitudes and economic necessity in Europe will show this.

Since modern history began the inhabitants of Europe have been divided into three classes. The manual workers, the priests and scholars, and the nobility. For the manual worker, peasant or artisan, work and a livelihood have always been closely connected. Whether they were tillers of the soil, the primary producers, or engaged in some other handicraft, there was a direct relationship between their work and the return in food or money. The lazy man either had to marry an industrious wife or become a beggar—or starve. In any case he was looked upon with disapproval, as a drag on the community, held up to scorn, and left as near starvation as communal feeling would allow. Children in the same way were trained to work as early as possible so that they might make their contribution. When work was done, if there was any energy left over, it was expended in dancing, feasting and merry-making—and the violence of country dances and country sports matched the type of energy that the farmer was accustomed to use in his ordinary working life.

All this was clear. The priest and scholar was in a more difficult position. He did not work directly at the production of food or commodities ; he expected to be supplied with these by a community to which he gave something yet more valuable. It depended on the priest and the state of mind of his parish, whether his contribution was highly esteemed. In Piers Plowman *Sloth* is the universal name for the parson ; but a parish priest in a remote Worcestershire village was perhaps hardly the best of his class. The priest should perhaps be judged by the best examples and the theory that lay behind the profession. Ideally the priest, scholar, doctor, lawyer, are learned and devoted men. They work, not with their hands, but their brains, and they devote the results of their study to the benefit of their fellow-men who have not the time or skill to study these subjects. In order to become expert in these matters a child must be taken young, taught certain things, and helped to learn how to perform the difficult mental operations neces-sary. Not all children are capable of them—just as not all children can draw—and very few are capable of them unless they are taught to perform them from an early age. Thus the learned class are workers in their own way, and are taught to work from quite early childhood.

The great difference between them and the peasant lies in the method by which they are rewarded. The peasant is rewarded very simply. If he ploughs five acres of land his corn crop, supposing the weather is kind, is five times as large as if he ploughed one acre. There is no such obvious return for the priest or scholar. He is dependent, for one thing, on the tastes of the public. A lifetime spent editing the text of the *Fathers* can receive no direct reward such as comes to the ploughman. The author may even receive nothing. There are probably as many hours of labour expended on a novel that can find no publisher as on a best-seller. Further, those who most need the services of priest, scholar, lawyer, doctor, are often least able to pay for them. The poor man with numberless children, the tenant turned out of his holding, the widow dying alone, all make a claim that the rich, powerful and happy do not. There has thus grown up among the members of this class a certain standard of public service, and this has been strengthened by the influence of the church. It was long ago realized that it was better for the priest to be " poor " and to receive the least rather than the greatest possible reward for his services. As the other professions grew up partly under the influence of the church, the professional man has traditionally been of moderate means. Teachers have never been thought worthy of very high rewards by the community, nothing like so high as managers of departments in big shops. Doctors and lawyers, though their standard of living is higher, are not *rich* men ; they regularly give a considerable amount of their services free to needy persons. They would never think of holding the community to ransom by a strike, though the doctors did once nearly threaten one.[1] The habits and ideas of work are thus taught to the pro-fessional classes from childhood, and unless a child does work, and work hard, all through the period of his

[1] Over Lloyd George's Health Insurance Act.

education he never learns enough to become a member of this body.

The aristocracy and the very rich are in a different category. Throughout mediæval Europe the lord was the fighting man, the leader of his own particular little army. He and his soldiers were supported by the peasants and artisans, prayed for by the priest, and justified these attentions by keeping peasant and priest safe from attack. This was the theory. But the lords fought for other motives than self-defence, and brought strife into districts where none need have been. It is curious how the mentality of petty nobles has descended to many of the politicians of to-day.

The fighting man did not work. He had no time and no need. He could take what he wanted, so that when he was not learning his trade, or hunting or jousting to keep his hand in, he was feasting or making love. As the centuries passed the position of the king and his nobles became more and more absurd. Some specialized in war such as Frederick the Great and brought destruction on themselves and their neighbours. Others lived lives of pleasure in a complete absence of serious business. When this was carried to such excess, as in the France of Louis XVI that the whole country was threatened with bankruptcy, the nation rose against this dangerous anachronism. No political revolution, however, could remove the real cause of the trouble: a class which had no necessity to work and had had no training in altruistic effort. In England of the eighteenth century the gentleman, as represented by Jane Austen, had nothing to do and no incentive to do it. There were no careers open to him but the church or the army. He could spend his time like Mr. Bennett " reading " in his library, or he could get drunk, make foolish wagers and gamble like the young Virginian. To have an uncle who was a lawyer was an almost fatal disgrace, and if a gentleman lost all his money the best thing he could do was to turn highwayman. If viewed from this standpoint most of the literature dealing with this period makes gloomy reading. The tradition flowed on to the next century. The Royal Dukes, sons of George III, were a group of men, some of fair ability, who were kept half occupied, without standards of conduct, and so passed much of their too abundant leisure in debauchery.

In the eighteenth century the tone of society was on the whole set by the aristocracy. Happiness and enjoyment were the lot of those who had no work to do. The tradition has lingered. In America, when oil was found in Oklahama on land given to the Indians as a reserve, the money was paid to the Indians. It was spent in riding about the country in Lincolns.[1] So in England recently the winner of a large sweepstake prize spent it in car rides and getting drunk in exactly the same manner—only he killed himself more rapidly than the Indians do. The unsatisfactory nature of the ideal is that a life of this kind, apart from its effect on the health, leaves the liver restless. His first idea is to drink alcohol as a means of staying the restlessness, and the Bright Young Things of to-day, who are essentially an unoccupied class, drink far more than their sisters and brothers in regular work ; and for just the same reason that all unoccupied people have drunk through English history. Then when alcohol fails to still the restlessness permanently, the man turns to speed. To-day he drives a fast car, in the past he hunted ; and the combination of horses and port was the characteristic life of the country gentleman for generations.

With the nineteenth century a complete change took place. The Reform Bill of 1832 destroyed the political preeminence of the aristocracy, and with political power the ideas of the middle classes became predominant. The rich men who took power in England from 1832 onwards were essentially members of the peasant class who had made great fortunes out of the industrial revolution without an essential change of ideal. They were not members of the priestly and professional class with their ideas of intangible value—such as learning—or their tradition of service to the lowest in the community. They were men who were accustomed to think in terms of the direct equivalence between effort and reward, and to count so many hours at the desk the equivalent of so much money or goods. For them the less successful members of their own class who still hauled weights or watched machines had their value assessed in

[1] The American equivalent of Rolls-Royces.

hours of work and expenditure of effort. There was no doubt whatever in the minds of the economists who described this state of things. Man worked for a livelihood. If he did not work he starved—and that was all there was to it. The aim of all employers therefore was to produce such conditions that men worked. Low wages forced a man to work continually, the refusal of parish relief, if a man's wife and children were not employed, forced the wife and children to work too. The employer who made others work worked himself. All England worked and Dr. Samuel Smiles applauded it.

From this period date theories of play. The surprised philosopher saw children *playing*. "Playing," he said. "Why are they not working? How can all this effort be dissipated on such frivolous objects when it might be devoted to securing the good of mankind." Amazed, almost scandalized, they invented theories to account for this levity. The most tragic of these theories is that play takes place when a child has any surplus energy, any that has not been squeezed out of him by work, and to read the writers you would think there was not much left.

"Theories of play" always seem a little ridiculous to our ears. Of course children play—so do adults. We are coming to ask rather, why do they work. It is this attitude which makes it important for schools and industry to-day to consider the real motives for effort, either in play or work.

In the first place the distinction between play and work must be removed. When work was unpleasant, done purely for money or to avoid punishment, then the distinction was obvious enough. It is still sufficiently obvious under certain circumstances to-day. But the unpleasantness of work and the disorder of play are both decreasing, and it is often difficult to draw a clear distinction between willing work and orderly, purposeful play. That distinction away, some things are clear.

(1) That the natural state of children and most adults is one of activity. What a person does depends on his powers. A small child, whose capacities for action are small, will satisfy his desire for activity by running round and round the room. The running is quite purposeless, and when the

child gets tired of going in one direction he turns and runs in the other.

> A cheerful old bear at the zoo
> Said I never have time to feel blue,
> When things feel a bit slow
> As I walk to and fro,—
> I reverse and proceed fro and to.

An older child, in the same state, gets her skipping-rope and skips. A still older child goes out and plays football, rides his cycle round the field, reads a book, or plays with plasticine. An adult who has no pressing duty to perform reads, writes letters, mends the furniture, tinkers with his car, or knits a jumper, or plays bridge. The activity in all cases serves the same purpose. It fills the mind and prevents the painful restlessness of idleness. It " passes the time ".

(2) Most people, children or adults, are kept from having to find too much personal amusement by their " work " For several hours a day they are at school or at some place of employment or engaged in the home. In most cases they are earning their living, or helping in some way to earn it. This activity is motivated by the most primitive of human instincts, and is specialized, as we pointed out before, in accordance with the custom of society. In addition to the motive of earning one's own living there is often the added incentive provided by a wife and children. The effort that these two impulses provide is very great and supplies the driving power when the desire for activity flags through fatigue, or when we suffer from a monotony that would make us vary our activity in a manner not approved of by our employers.

It is when activity is pursued under full compulsion that it becomes " work " in the worst sense, and it is more often the conditions than the activity itself that cause the necessity for compulsion. In the first place there is fatigue. If work or play is continued beyond a certain time fatigue sets in ; and what was a perfectly pleasant activity becomes work that we only do because we fear the consequences of a refusal to continue. Closely related to fatigue due to length of period is restlessness or fatigue due to bad conditions, defective ventilation, excessive heat or cold, ugly, squalid surroundings. Next a sense of unwillingness arises when none of our instinctive sources of energy is tapped. If we are working for our own advantage we find the work easy—if we know that however hard we work we shall only get our stated wage, and that smaller than we think it ought to be, then we grow weary of working for another, and long to be home digging our own vegetable patch or engaged in some other activity for our own good. Further, if our work demands no specialized skill in which we take a pride, we shall grow weary of it and long for the hours when we can do woodwork or mend our motor-cycle. Again, we resent work when some of our strongest impulses are denied satisfaction during the period. Thus a girl longs for the time to come when she can leave the factory and meet her young man.

All this is very important in dealing with children in school. There is no doubt that most children nowadays enjoy school, and if they call what they do there " work ", feel for that work no particular distaste. That was not so in the past. The subjects that the children are taught are in many cases the same, but the whole conditions and methods of teaching are different. For one thing great care is taken not to weary the children. There are opportunities for recreation and movement and frequent changes of lesson. That has removed one of the great obstacles to learning. Then the conditions such as ventilation, heating, light, space are all becoming more pleasant, and the teachers themselves are continually trying to make the children happy. Lastly, the curriculum is wider, so that many of the things children want to do, such as dancing, singing, games and nature study can now be done in school better than away from it. There are thus to-day fewer of the reasons for disliking " work " in school and wishing to be free of it.

Although there is a readiness for activity the ordinary conditions of work to-day are such that natural activity would not lead men to do *all* that is required of them. Nor would it lead children to learn all that they should know. In the past fear has regularly been used to supply the necessary extra energy. If this is to be abandoned it is necessary to think of other incentives to effort.

Far the best is, of course, an understanding of the necessity for the work. We are then able to rely on the full force of an innate tendance. We must plough the land or starve, pump the ship or sink, or, in less dramatic circumstances, get a trousseau finished, or our sweet-pea seeds set. Children, as has been said before, can be got to respond to purposes that are more or less immediate, and the more closely these purposes touch their deepest interest the more vigour they will expend in realizing them.

The U.S.S.R. relies on this understanding of purpose as a stimulant to much of the effort of its subjects. The attempt to establish cities and airports in the far north of Siberia is one fraught with hard work of the dreariest kind, yet it is willingly undertaken and faithfully performed by men and women who believe in the end that is to be accomplished. The development of the country, the victory over a hostile environment, the securing of national prosperity and national safety all seem worth the effort to achieve them.

With children or less intelligent people there is need of further incentives ; and perhaps the chief of them is praise. When the food shortage in Moscow was at its height, a certain collective farm raised a very fine herd of pigs. These were sent to the city with their herdsmen. Pigs and wardens were met at the station and marched through the streets with a brass band. There is an element of comedy in this, but the principle is sound. In many works this method is carried further, and possibly made more effective, by the addition of a cash bonus.

Much the same principle applies in the development in any individual of a sense of skill and pride in his competence. On the whole the exercise of any skilled function is pleasant. We like doing anything that we think we do well. It is extraordinary how quickly a child will respond to this. Let him once find that he can do sums and he will enjoy doing them. In the same way a skilled workman enjoys the practice of his craft even though after a time he grows tired and wishes for some other form of activity. Yet he is hardly ever too tired to be lured into giving a demonstration of his skill, and will voluntarily work overtime in order to finish something in which he takes particular pride.

Of the same type of incentive is competition. Schools use it, and over-use it. Without adopting a high moral attitude it is possible to disapprove, faintly, of school competition. It is a motive to which only some children respond, and it is one of which people rapidly tire. Some small reward to *everybody* who achieves a certain standard is a far better incentive.

In addition to all this the worker or child at school finds himself part of a group engaged in a common pursuit. His gregarious impulses are called into play. Most people, unless they work under very bad conditions, feel this "loyalty" and sense of the group to which they belong. "My school", says the teacher. "Our place", says the workman. In districts where there are very small businesses producing high-grade work the sense of community among the workers is strong. The attitude of the Birmingham jeweller is typical. Much of the best work is done by firms that only employ half a dozen people, and their workers are all highly skilled. In addition to the personal pride and self-respect that the man has in his own ability there is also the pride in the organization of which he is no inconsiderable part. On the other hand, such is the adaptability of human nature, some people like belonging to a large organization. They get a thrill of pride as their personality expands to include the whole. In their work they find companionship and often friendship, and a most satisfying sense of social solidarity.

One of the commonest charges thrown about at staff meetings when students or children are under discussion is that So-and-So is lazy. The charge is usually quite unjustified. That So-and-So does her needlework badly cannot be doubted, but the explanation may be something quite different from laziness. The defect may be due to ill-health, worry, or over-work, all of which things produce a lessening of effort in all or some directions. It may be due to inability or extreme distaste for the subject, or it may be due to some rival interest such as a love affair. There is no doubt that some people possess more disposable energy than others, and the less energy a person has the lazier he seems to be to more energetic neighbours. It is also true that different people have different scales of value and that what seems tremendously important to a teacher of mathematics seems contemptible to Smith minor determined to get into the cricket XI. Laziness as a school sin, is far less frequent than it is supposed to be and needs investigating rather than immediate condemnation and " disciplinary measures ". As an industrial sin it is far more often due to the organization than to the badness of the individual.

There is an interesting combination of all these motives to effort called ambition. It is of course a virtue. Ambition is to be prepared to sacrifice all that can be sacrificed without loss of honour, e.g. your wife's happiness and your children's affection, to making money and position. The man of ambition wants to be rich, to be looked up to, to hold power and influence, and of course to benefit his state and nation. The man of ambition is prepared to work hard, to deny himself pleasures, and to sacrifice his life if need be to the glorious goal of his own advancement. It is an urge compounded of some of the strongest emotions, and it is differentiated from the ordinary main desire to earn a living by the enormous strength of self-assertion involved, and the unshakable belief that you alone and your own wishes are truly worthy of consideration. What you have to give is unique, and you are justified in taking any steps to ensure that you are in a position to give it. A grateful nation will doubtless bury you in Westminster Abbey. In its less extreme form it is a variant of competition and schools encourage it, as they encourage competition, as a cheap and easy form of incentive. They offer certain positions of authority and certain rewards. The attainment of them may have good or bad results, and the ambitious boy is generally only admirable when his ambition is kept within reasonable limits. Why a " man's ambition " should have become a sentimental theme, especially with dramatists, is hard to see. It is the satisfaction of an impulse, as good or bad, certainly no better, than a " woman's love " that is regularly sacrificed to it.

If these are the advantages of work, unemployment brings a complicated series of evils in its train. This has of recent years been realized by social workers. It is not only the loss of money, though that is serious enough. It is the loss of opportunities for activity and interest, the loss of companionship, and the loss of the sense of social solidarity. A man at work has a place in the structure of society, a part in its purposes. A man out of work has none. A few men, when out of work, devise amusements for themselves. One shop assistant went off on a cycle tour through Wales. Many, if they can, take to working on allotments. Almost all, if provided with an opportunity, take part in social activities and manual work. The unemployed man, lounging unhappily at the street corner, demonstrates more clearly than anything else the human need of activity and purpose.

It has been shown by many of the modern schools where the child is not forced to do anything, as well as by the Russian Prison camps that people, after a time, would rather work than do nothing. It is claimed, and we can well believe it, that a child after being left to wander about by himself comes and asks to be taught. Certainly many children, from the age of three upwards, insist on being sent to school. They are dissatisfied with the unco-ordinated activities of the nursery and crave the stimulus and companionship of school life. No child who is properly taught should regard school as an infliction. On the other hand, as was said before we generally need from child or worker just a little more effort than he is prepared voluntarily to give. The great problem is how to get the extra effort in the most satisfactory way. The ultra-modern school in its exaggerated search for freedom does not realize this. It is so engaged in attacking all other schools where any form of incentive is used that it forgets to use any itself. One such school, boasting of its academic successes, proudly stated that one of its children had passed matriculation at 18. If that boy wishes to take up any scholarly profession he will curse the laxity of his education and the waste of time. Of another it was stated that he had gloriously achieved the job of a chauffeur to a lady of fortune. It appears from other statements that the boy was clever. He too, when he considers the prospects open to him, will not be very satisfied with his preparation for life.

That we use incentives to work need not mean tyranny nor a repression of the child's natural wishes. Children are unstable and they know little of the world. The rôle of the adult is to help them to overcome the defects of their immaturity. Children as a whole welcome this help, and feel that they have been defrauded if they do not receive it. A class of children will protest bitterly if they are left without supervision. " We didn't *want* to rag but we couldn't help it " is a complaint that is made by boys of 10 or 11. There is no doubt that some children are made by the examination system to work too hard, but in many cases they are their own taskmasters and need to be discouraged rather than over encouraged to work. It is also true that some children are so badly taught that they dislike work, but this number is constantly diminishing. In any well run school to-day the children find a real freedom rather than repression in the encouragement and incentives to work.

FOR DISCUSSION

1.—Recall your own schooldays. What repression did you suffer, if any—and what forms of incentives were used ?
2.—What means of keeping children happily occupied would you recommend outside school hours ?
3.—What do you think about homework ? Do you agree with those who wish to abolish it ?
4.—Discuss examinations as an incentive to work.
5.—Study the activities of a domestic cat or dog. For about what proportion (of time) is the animal active and for what proportion asleep or resting.
6.—If you were quite free of the necessity of earning your living how would you spend your time.

BOOKS

JANE AUSTEN, *Pride and Prejudice*
THACKERAY, *The Virginians*
DEFOE, *Moll Flanders*   Aspects of the eighteenth and
R. FULFORD, *Royal Dukes*   early nineteenth.
FIELDING, *Tom Jones*
Voyage of the " Chelyuskin ". Russian ideas.
S. and B. WEBB, *Soviet Communism, a New Civilization*, esp. Ch. ix. and xii.
H. G. WELLS, *The Work, Wealth and Happiness of Mankind*, Ch. viii.
A. S. NEILL, *A Dominie in Doubt.*
        A Dominie Dismissed.

PART II

THE TOOLS OF MIND

CHAPTER XII

SENSATION AND PERCEPTION

" Both what they half perceive and half create.*"*

In a previous section of this book it was shown how purposeful man's activities are, and how it is impossible to explain impulses and actions except in terms of purpose. The same thing applies to thought and other intellectual processes. Mental processes can be *described* without reference to purpose, but we cannot *understand* them unless we also consider the part that they play in the economy of life. In considering this it will become clear that many apparently simple functions are very complicated and have been devised to fit a peculiar need with great nicety. The most striking example of this accurate adjustment is afforded by perception.

The basis of all our knowledge is supplied by our contact, through the senses, with the world around us ; but this contact is by no means direct or simple. The first distinction to be made is that between *sensation* and *perception*. The former is what we actually experience at the moment, the latter is the *interpretation* of that experience in the light of our previous experience.

It is almost impossible to describe a pure sensation. An adult practically never has one—and, if he had, he would have difficulty in discovering words in which to describe it. As good an account as is possible of the distinction between sensation and perception is contained in this account of a

149

recovery from a fainting fit. " I saw in front of me something red with black bars across it, and after I had been looking at it for some time I realized that it was the fire in the grate that I saw ". Even in this case the sensation was not quite pure—the word " bars " introduces an idea which could not have been apprehended by sensation alone, but the transition from the sensation of black and red to the interpretative *perception* of the fire is well marked. If we could see the visual world simply as colour, without shape or line or distance, then we should have a pure sensation of it ; what we actually see is given us by perception which interprets the different colours as meaning light and shade, buildings and sky, men, now near, now afar off.

This interpretation is made on the basis of past experience. We have had sensations from the different senses all arising from the same thing. We have *seen* our pen and *felt* it in our hand, we have *seen* a hen and *heard* her cluck, or attempted to catch the moon and failed to reach her. We do not forget such experiences altogether, and thus we come to give *meaning* to the different separate sense impressions which we receive.

It is argued by some modern psychologists that the attempt to base our knowledge of objects on the result of experience is a mistake. If we did not first distinguish an object how could we have experience of it. All our sense experience—in its physical form—is continuous : colour beside colour, sound after sound, and at some point this experience is broken up into visual objects, or the sound of a voice discriminated from the background of general noise. Koehler [1] maintains that the division of direct sense experience into objects is as primitive as the experience itself. When once the division has taken place then other qualities can be added to the object thus discriminated by association from the other senses. This seems true. It certainly meets the difficulty of the beginning of the process of analysis. James suggests that to the baby the universe is a big, blooming, buzzing confusion. He fails to offer any adequate explanation of the *first* moments when objects become discriminated.

In our sense-knowledge of the world lies one of the greatest

[1] *Gestalt Psychology.*

marvels of psychology or any other science. We do not come into contact with any object directly. There is little doubt that we perceive through the instrumentality of the brain, and the brain is shut off from the world in a hard, bony box, packed in carefully with membranes and fluid and connected with the exterior of the body only by long filaments of a particular construction which are called nerves, and which look something like threads of dirty white cotton. Along these nerves pass impulses which may be chemical or electrical in character ; these impulses go to the brain and we see, or hear or touch. As far as any man can understand there is no common quality between change of electrical potential in a nerve and a view of an almond tree in full bloom against a blue sky, or a similar change in another nerve and the hearing of the " Unfinished Symphony " ; yet the only *direct* antecedent to these sense impressions of colour or sound is a change in a nerve, and the transition from one to the other remains an unfathomable mystery.

Each of us at each moment of sensation creates the world anew. A slight change in our sense organs or brain, and the world, for us, is different. For those born colour blind the world lacks a decoration that it possesses for other men ; the deaf live in a world which is different from that enjoyed by those with hearing, and, for all we know, each of us experiences a world considerably different from that of his fellow men. There can be no doubt whatever that in certain ways each of us lives in a world which is peculiar to himself. No two men have absolutely identical senses. One can see colours in a shadowed rock which another cannot see, and some folk can catch the separate notes of an orchestra which are to others mere noise. As Quoodle, in Mr. Chesterton's *Flying Inn*, remarks :

> They haven't got no noses,
> Those fallen sons of Eve.

and the " noselessness of man " must be a marvel to any intelligent dog.

The wonder of all this should be increased when we come to consider the highly complicated mechanism of any one sense organ. The eye for example is very similar to a camera with a diaphragm (the iris), a lens, and a sensitive plate (the retina). This is all well known. The light passes through the hole in the iris (the pupil), is focussed by the lens, and the retina is stimulated and sends impulses through the optic nerve to the brain. If the light is bright, the pupil is contracted; if dim, expanded. This can be seen very well in cats and can be observed also in men. The lens is also capable of accommodation according to the distance of the object regarded, the curvature of the lens being controlled by the ciliary muscle by means of which it is suspended. With a little practice one can feel this accommodation on turning the eyes to a near object.

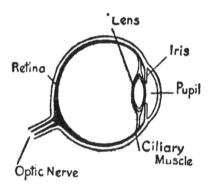

Further, the retina is not all equally sensitive, and in each eye there is a blind spot just where the optic nerve enters the eye. We are never conscious of this blind patch unless we use some special experiment such as the following to demonstrate it.

Place the two thumbs together, look steadily at the left one with the right eye (the left eye being shut), and move the right thumb slowly away. At one point, usually when the thumbs are about four inches apart, the right thumb will vanish and almost immediately reappear. It vanishes from sight at the moment when the rays from it are focussed on the blind spot in the retina of the eye. There is yet a further complication; we have two eyes and the nerves from them, so far from uniting and going to one place in the brain, go to the two different hemispheres, yet we see *one* world. Only in abnormal conditions do we see double!

The delicate adjustment of iris or lens, and the supplementing of experience to fill up the blind spot, go on for us all the time, and we do not usually give any conscious attention to them. However, we are not unaffected by them since we make judgments on the basis of them. For instance, it is mainly the movement of convergence and the slight difference in retinal images from the two eyes which enable us to judge distance. Cover one eye and try to put your finger on a spot ; it is difficult to be swift and accurate. People who have only one eye learn to use other indications as a means of judging distance, but the normal person with two eyes relies on those given above.

Our sense experience itself is thus a very complicated thing, but it is only the basis of perception ; we at once pass beyond it to something else, and are normally interested in these sensations, not for themselves, but as the sign of some object, which we think of as being external to, and independent of ourselves, not as being the product of our brain taking its cue from certain changes in the nerves. An illustration from sound and sight combined will make this clear. Suppose we are watching a sea with breaking waves, and follow up a wave as it comes towards the shore. At first it is an irregular line in the sea, lighter on one side than the other, green or blue according to the day. At a certain point it changes shape and colour, the sound it makes is altered and we say that the wave has " broken ". Our *sensations* are visual and auditory, and through these sensations we can *perceive* that the wave has broken, although we attend comparatively little to the actual sensations we experience.

Unless we have a special aim in observing, we are apt not to attend to sensations in a discriminating way at all. The artist attends directly to visual impressions, the musician to sounds, the poet to emotions, but the average man sees a breaking wave, hears a stream, or feels gloomy. The sensation is recognized as the sign of some thing or condition to which we pay attention while the sensation itself may be disregarded.

In some cases we get this interpretation carried even further. In the case of the wave it is the external object which provides the sensations directly, in other cases this is not so. If a man is looking over an estuary from the headland he may say, " Oh, yes, I can see the bar." What he actually sees is a line of breakers near the mouth of the estuary, but that line of foam means for him the presence of shallow water—i.e., the bar—and the sense experience of certain colours and shapes is interpreted directly as this.

This process of interpretation can be carried even further in the intellectual sphere. Much of our thought consists of making one thing mean another. One of the most complete examples is afforded by this page. Certain marks on paper cause certain visual sensations to the reader. These sensations are interpreted as words, really vocal sounds, these sounds stand for certain things or ideas ; yet when we read, the ideas alone are really present to our minds, and we cease to pay attention to the various sense impressions which are for us the source of the ideas presented through them. Almost exactly the same result would be achieved if this book were written in French, or any other language with which we are well acquainted.

Much of the difficulty of learning to draw is caused by this tendency to objectify sensations. Very few people, without training, attend to what they actually see. They are too pre-occupied with the object that the sensations stand for, to realize the sensations themselves. Children's drawings illustrate this clearly. It is very hard to get them to look at the object. They glance at it just sufficiently to see that it is, say, a green bottle that they are to draw, and then they proceed to draw the bottle, more or less accurately, according to the idea of green bottles already present in their minds. This idea will generally not include the peculiar qualities of the bottle set up for the model, so that the particular shape, or the high lights on the glass, or anything like realistic variations of colour are not present.

The history of art affords interesting examples of the attempt to isolate different aspects of sense experience. Early art, such as Greek vase paintings, shows little knowledge of perspective. The drawings are so treated that they could be turned directly into low relief, and it is the influence of sculpture that is strongest in the arrangement of forms. In the later vases there is an attempt to represent scenes in three dimensions and therefore some perspective is needed.

The most obvious of the sense differences between near and far objects is seized upon, and figures more remote are represented *higher up* in the picture, though, as they are all equally men, they remain the same size. When the Italian artists of the school of Giotto attempt to show perspective they nearly always commit faults which result in the picture seeming to go rapidly up hill. This is very obvious in some interiors, as in the *Annunciation* of Fra Angelico. On the other hand in larger landscape pictures such as the *Procession of Lorenzo the Magnificent*, many devices are employed.

The more distant figures are made smaller and they are set upon hills, but in spite of this the artist has not achieved any illusion because he has not observed the effects of atmosphere, and in his painting the remote figures are as *sharp* as those close at hand and the colours are as clear. Modern perspective is an extremely complicated thing, including arrangements of lines, difference in size and position of objects, and changes in colour and distinctness. Now that visual sensations have been analysed, it is easy for a student to pick up at least the rudiments of perspective in a short time, but it took centuries of thought by the ablest artists before this analysis was accomplished.

A further analysis was achieved by the Impressionists some years ago, when they demonstrated that a colour which seems one is not one, but a number of colours, and that the most effective method of painting a shadow which seems grey, may be to put on reds, blues and greens pure, and allow them to mix " in the eye " itself. Yet another element is now being isolated from a general sense experience —the emotion that accompanies it—and some modern cubist artists claim to present this emotion, while disregarding the exact forms and colours in the object presented.

The interpretation of sense impressions is perception. And this interpretation, nearly universal as it is, is also complicated and contains many elements. We realize that if we study for ourselves the details of a common act of perception. If we see an object on a table and perceive that it is a glass of milk, our visual sensations are complicated and are further supplemented by memories, however faint, of past sensations derived from other senses. We " perceive ", apparently directly, by sight alone, that the glass is hard and smooth and cold, and we perceive this without touching the glass. This is because we have connected certain remembered sensations of touch with certain visual appearances. We also perceive that the milk is liquid and cold, and, in so far as we know that it is milk, that it has a certain taste. Anything unusual in the taste would be perceived as contrary to expectation, e.g., if the milk was sour, had been boiled, or contained glycerine. All the knowledge that we have of a glass of milk is really called up by the sight of it, and would become operative if circumstances demanded it. We know that milk quenches thirst, is a food, will spill if the glass is tipped, and will help to take out ink stains. The sight of the glass of milk does not call up the thought of all these qualities consciously, but our knowledge of them all is implicit in our behaviour towards the milk, and is implied when we speak of the liquid as " milk ". The same thing applies when we call the container a glass. The use of the words " milk " and " glass " enables us to sum up and distinguish many varied experiences of taste, sight, touch and use, and to refer to this whole mass of qualities without the labour of individual specification.

Every known object in our experience is thus built up of memories of experiences from the different senses, and any one single experience may call up the whole complex or group of experiences. Thus a red glow on the floor suggests at once fire, something alight and burning. A certain smell tells us at once of new cakes for tea. We see a gleam on the road and know that it is wet. Sight is the sense which we use most in this way, because we apprehend more things by sight than we do by any other sense, but we can experience the same thing in regard to hearing. If we lie in bed sick and listen to the noises of the house and the street, each sound carries its meaning. The rattle is Jane stoking the fire, that clatter is Tom tobogganing downstairs on a tray, that purr is a Daimler car, that scraping is Mr. Brown's dog trying to get the gate open. The nature of the interpretation of sounds is made startlingly evident if we suffer from a temporary deafness. We can then hear sounds, but in an unusual guise, so that we cannot bring our past experience to bear on their interpretation.

Smell must be as important to an animal as sight and

hearing are to us. A kitten will *smell* for its dinner all over a sheet of *The Times* spread on the floor, and regularly smells a chair before sitting down on it ; in both those cases a man looks. To some men, as to Shelley, smell is more important than it is to others, but for all normal people the easiest way to find out what is in a jam pot is to smell it, and chemists regularly identify many substances in this way.

We form a percept of an object, then, when we give meaning to a sense impression, using remembered sense impressions to help our interpretation. We can go farther and construct a " concept " of something which has no concrete existence—of " a teacher " in general, as distinguished from the particular examples about us, or of " Justice ", as distinguished from particular acts of justice or injustice. All this will be referred to again in the chapters on words and thought, but an example from two particularly striking concepts is worth giving, in order to show to what extent we can pass beyond sense impressions which we yet regard as indicating the thing conceived. Time and space are not apprehended directly, though we usually think that they are. " Time " is an elaborate judgment based on the fact that one event follows another, and that certain synchronizations are possible. We use clocks now habitually and we learn roughly how many events can occur in a space of clock time, i.e., while the hands of a clock move a certain distance ; but, because we judge time in hours or minutes, this does not mean that the flight of time always appears constant to us. Some hours go very fast, others very slowly, and, if we had no external means to aid us, we should be hard put to it to estimate periods of duration. There is no direct experience of time, but only a judgment based on a rough estimate of the number of events that take place, while certain other events occur. When we wait five minutes for a desired person to arrive, the five minutes seem half an hour. But half an hour of interesting talk seems but five minutes. In the same way there is no direct experience of space. When we perceive space visually we connect visual impressions with images of movement. As we develop, we compare a visual impression, not with the image of the movements necessary to reach it, but with a standard which derives its meaning from such images, though when we use

157

the standard we do not necessarily call up the images. For instance, we look at a distant hill and say that it looks five miles away. The meaning to be attached to the scale of miles is a kinæsthetic one and is based on movement ; a mile is 2000, or so, paces. In actual fact the meaning of " five miles " will differ in different circumstances. If we are young and strong it may be a pleasant distance for a walk, if we are getting on in years it may be a prohibitive distance, if we have a car it may be a mere nothing—a few minutes' run.

Besides visual, we have auditory space—we locate sounds, and here, too, the basis of the judgment of space is the connection of a sound and the performance of certain movements to bring us into relation with its source. We never perceive space itself any more than we perceive time itself ; we only see objects in a special arrangement or make certain movements and reach certain goals. These two concepts are built up from our experience, but are not directly given by it.

The tendency, then is for the mind to interpret sense impressions as being certain objects, and to attend to these objects rather than to the sense impressions which form our direct knowledge of them. The utility of this course is clear. We act on, and are affected by our environment, and it is more convenient to react promptly to " objects " than to be concerned with our sensations. What is important to us is that milk is good to drink. It is of far less moment to us that, as the glass now stands, there are interesting reflections from the white milk on to the dark polished table. We also interpret our sense impressions as indications of qualities in persons or things, just as much as indications of the things themselves. A certain expression on a person's face means that he is angry or pleased, and we say that we " *saw* his anger ". So, too, movements may be interpreted as motives. Such a phrase as " I saw he meant to strike me " is quite common. We do not, of course, see his intention to strike, we see certain movements which we interpret as indications of his intention. There is an obvious utility in our paying attention directly to the meanings of what we see and hear from people. We need to anticipate the action of others so as to aid or prevent them. The actual sense impressions on which we base our interpretation are comparatively unimportant, and we quickly learn to go beyond them to their meaning.

As the tendency of our thoughts is to interpret any sensation, we are most unwilling, generally, to leave any sensation unexplained. If on our wall we observe a lighter patch we nearly always start to investigate its cause. Is it damp? No, because the edges are ill defined instead of being marked by a line. Is it a difference in the paint? No, we should have seen it before. Is it a reflected light from some picture glass? We hold our hand just in front of it, there is a shadow. The problem is solved. If we hear a curious noise in our room we cannot rest till we have interpreted it by referring it to some cause. Sensations divorced from their meaning worry and annoy us.

This strong tendency to interpret often gives rise to illusions, especially when the sensations themselves are faint. These faint sensations tend to be interpreted in a way that fits in with their general setting or with our mood at the time. A sign-post standing on a bank above a road, may become for the belated and nervous traveller a white woman with a baby in her arms. The child whose imagination is obsessed with ogres sees strange faces in the flickering shadows that his candle throws on the ceiling. As a general rule those who expect ghosts see them, and all those who care to listen may hear phantom bells in the sea surge, or angel voices in the church chimes.

It would be a mistake to think that our perception is limited to the interpretation of isolated objects. It extends much farther, to whole situations. If we recognize any class of objects, horse, dog, or even, for a baby, a feeding-bottle, we have recognized not a particular thing, but a member of a class. We have performed an act of abstraction, and formed a scheme—an abstract scheme—and judged that this object is included in it. Thus a small child seeing for the first time a Bedlington Terrier makes a false identification and cries out,

" Look ! that lady has a *lamb* on a lead ! "

The child gets great pleasure from these identifications, especially when he is learning them and the words that describe them.

" Bow-wow ! " says the baby. " Haystack ! " says the slightly older child taken for a ride in a car and grins with pleasure. It is very difficult to discover exactly what qualities are accepted as the basis of these generalizations, but there is no doubt that the end of them is useful action.

Very rapidly the child goes farther, and reacts not only to the object but to the whole situation. A child seeing his mother with a cup and a spoon expresses lively satisfaction in the anticipation of being given orange juice, or he resists the whole situation that is leading up to going to bed. This understanding of the situation as a whole is also characteristic of the higher animals. An intelligent dog knows perfectly well what is meant when he is asked to " shake hands ", but he will only do it if you have a bit of biscuit available when you make your request.

The extent to which the *whole* situation influences action may be considered as one of the marks of intelligence. The situations with which the adult has to deal are often extremely complex, and the more intelligent the person is the more completely will he understand and respond to all the various factors. The important thing is that, as in the case of dog or haystack, we should see all the various elements in the situation as part of one whole—as part, in fact, of a scheme. For it is only if we have unified them into a scheme that we can deal with them by thought. We can see this in relation to memory. It is easy to remember a tune, that has a definite pattern, impossible to remember a number of unrelated notes. If we can group the figure of a telephone number according to some plan 1212 we can remember them, if they resist our attempts at grouping they will slip again and again from our mind. The abstraction and grouping of sense elements gives us our perception of the *thing*, the grouping of things and the abstraction of their common elements gives us the concept, and a further grouping and abstraction gives us the whole situation.

One of the modern developments in education and one which is particularly due to Madame Montessori, is sense training. The aim of such training is to make children discriminate between slightly different stimuli to the same sense organ and to attend to sense impressions as well as to the objects for which they stand. Madame Montessori's apparatus comprises coloured silks for discriminating colours, pieces of wood for telling weight, height, thickness, size and shape, sand paper and various materials for touch sensations, and whistles and bells for sound. The children arrange their bricks, place the insets in their correct places or handle the stuffs for some time before they are taught the names which correspond to the different sense impressions. This education of the senses has, she claims, many advantages. It lays the foundations of art and æsthetic appreciation. It is a source of pleasure to the individual, and develops refined senses which do not need the strong and gross stimulation that less delicate ones require. A man who has learnt to take delight in the changing greys of clouds and varying blues of shadows does not need the garish light of Piccadilly Circus to amuse him. Lastly, in many professions and trades, e.g. the medical, watch-making, milling and many others, a man needs refined senses and it is a waste of time and a danger to the community if all this sensory discrimination has to be acquired late in life.

In all this there is much truth and Madame Montessori is right when she claims that little children find the mere exercise of their senses interesting enough. But at the same time, sense training should not be regarded as an end in itself. Mere sense discrimination rapidly ceases to be interesting, it is important and interesting in connection with a purpose that lies beyond it. An adult does not take prolonged pleasure in discriminating shades of colour merely as shades, but when he wishes to paint a picture, or paper a room, the occupation becomes interesting. Even such an advertisement as the following may be fraught with the greatest interest for the reader who wants an " exact match " for her frock, and the effort to discriminate and remember the different shades may, in such a case, occupy all one's thought.

———'s Hosiery
In the newest shades——
Flesh, Nude, Sunburn, Sahara, Beige, Banana,
Sand, Putty, Skin, Peach, Black and White.

It is necessary, therefore, not only to train the senses so that the individual can find pleasure in the exercise of them, but also to connect sense-training with a purpose as early as possible, and to let the child discriminate colours in order to draw, or sounds in order to sing, or rhythm in order to dance to it. This would do away with much of the apathy or inertia which is too often seen in an infant school, where the little mites sit and look blankly at certain bricks on their desk, and have apparently no idea what to do next with them and no impulse to do anything.

Sense training may assist, but it cannot produce that much more valuable thing, observation. For " observation " we need not only to experience the sensation, but to make it a part of our general body of knowledge. We do this by reflecting on it. One of Madame Montessori's children one day looked up and cried, " Oh, the sky is blue ". He had not only had a sense impression (he had had that many times before), but he had made the present impression part of an organized group of things which were blue. Conan Doyle's *Sherlock Holmes* stories provide the most famous examples of observation. From a study of Holmes's methods it will become clear at once that it was fineness of sensation that made his observations possible ; but that this fine sense-development would have been useless without the power to select, interpret, and use his sense experiences. He did see a few more things than did the dull officers from Scotland Yard, but the great difference lay in his skill in selecting relevant details, and in the additional knowledge that he was able to use in their interpretation. It is easy for an expert to tell a man's profession by his hands, but for the inexperienced an obvious sign may not carry its meaning simply through ignorance. Most coal hewers have their hands bent to a certain shape through the use of the pick. One who had never been in a coal mining district might notice the shape of the hand and not know how to interpret it, and so the " observation " would be useless. It is study and experience rather than a refined sense training that produces true " observation ".

FOR DISCUSSION

1.—What types and methods of sense training are used in schools ? What do you consider their value to be ?
2.—Give a critical account of any " observation " lessons you have experienced. Do you think this a useful form of lesson ?

3.—Try to write an exact description of any event, e.g., the way a twig catches fire and burns (state whether the twig is wet or dry), or make a drawing of a breaking wave. In the latter case the position of sun (s), observer (o), wave (w), should be as under and the time about midday.

```
                    ————————w
        s
                        o
```

4.—Try again with the position as follows and the time evening:

```
            s
        ————————w
            o
```

See if you can recollect differences in the appearance of the wave. Remember that waves have shadows and reflections. State which details you mention are *memories* of sense impressions, and which are reasoned deductions.

5.—Give examples of occasions on which time seemed to pass unusually fast or unusually slowly. Can you explain the illusion in any of the cases you give ?

6.—When travelling in a tram-car or train, attempt to determine the professions or trades of your fellow passengers. Give the grounds for your decisions.

7.—Give a detailed account of an attempt made by you to interpret an unfamiliar sense experience.

8.—Collect from your reading in literature (prose and poetry) any strikingly accurate description of sensations. Refer especially to Keats' poetry.

9.—Give an example of a pleasurable and of a painful sense experience. Can you suggest what causes the pleasure or pain in each case ?

10.—Observe which sensations a baby seems to find most pleasing.

11.—On what occasions have you relied almost solely on visual sensation, on auditory sensation, on tactile sensation (touch), or on olfactory sensation (smell) for guidance ?

12.—Describe the methods by which the Boy Scout Troops try to make their members observant.

BOOKS

G. F. Stout, *Analytic Psychology.*
  Manual of Psychology. Bks. ii. and iii. Sensation and perception.
Madame Montessori, *The Montessori Method.* Ch. xii.–xiv. Sense training.
Brown Smith, *The Child Under Eight.*
Bone, *The Service of the Hand in School.*
Browning, *Fra Lippo Lippi.* The quarrel between realistic and symbolic art.
H. Sturt, *Principles of Understanding.*
Wolfgang Koehler, *Gestalt Psychology.*

CHAPTER XIII

ATTENTION AND INTEREST

By no endeavour
Can a magnet ever
Attract a Silver Churn !

PERCEPTION, as we have seen, is a very complex process resulting in the apprehension of an object which appears external to us, and has a unity and character of its own. This apprehension in ordinary circumstances appears extremely rapid, but it really occupies an appreciable extent of time. It is possible to expose an object for so brief a moment that perception cannot take place, partly because we cannot make the necessary eye accommodation, partly because the sensations caused by the object have not time to be interpreted. For full perception, therefore, we need to hold a sense impression before our minds for a certain space of time, and this holding of a sense impression in thought is generally called attending to it, and *attention* is the name for the process. In ordinary, and particularly in educational use, attention is used of something much more protracted. A fraction of a second's attention will allow us to perceive an object. When we speak of attention in the usual way, we mean that the object has occupied our minds for minutes or hours. It is this prolonged attention which is the subject of this chapter.

Like other developed mental powers, attention has its origin in very simple forms of instinctive behaviour. In the chapters on instincts it was pointed out that an instinct has three parts, the cognitive, the affective, and the conative. The developments of the affect were treated in the chapter on emotion ; conation was shown to develop into will ; the cognitive part of the instinct is the primitive form of attention. Before we can feel an emotion or perform an action we must apprehend a situation ; as soon as an emotion has been aroused and action has started, we continue to be absorbed in our course of conduct, we are interested in it, and attend to it. For example, if we meet a pretty baby we stop and look at it, may stretch out a finger for it to grasp, or, if we are privileged, take it in our arms. During all this time we attend to the baby. A young man turns round and looks after a girl who has " caught his eye ". So, too, we can be " fascinated " by some object of terror and quite unable to withdraw our attention from it. Any natural stimulant to an instinct will catch and hold our attention for a time, and we describe the state of mind thus produced by saying that we are interested in the object. Attention and interest are naturally aroused by the same object ; it is only under more developed conditions that we get a partial divorce between attention and interest.

If we wish, therefore, to know what are the natural objects of interest and attention, we must look to the instincts. We can see this very clearly in the case of a cat. Any small moving object will attract it, but of all its toys it loves best a celluloid ball which rolls so lightly that it mimics the movements of a living animal, or a real bird's feather, which still smells of a natural object of prey. It is curious to see how the cat's attitude changes when the circumstances nearly approach his normal hunting. A marble lying on the carpet is not a bad toy, but when that marble rolls into a hole then the cat becomes enthralled, sits and watches the crack, reaches for the marble with his paw, and may spend a quarter of an hour in attempts to elicit the marble, which he disregards when it is once more lying on the open carpet.

With children the development of the different instincts is marked by the growth of new interests. A small baby can attend to little beyond his food, and his interest is centred in his bottle or his mother's breast ; one slightly older attends to the movements of people and things about him : mud-pies and brick-building have their turn, and later the interests of the hunting life. Later still, the young man develops an interest in the opposite sex and a pretty girl holds his attention. Then, later still, a home and family occupy his mind, and the business or profession which makes these possible.

In the adult man it is by no means so clear that all his interests spring from instincts. There are certainly many in which the connection is by no means direct. In some cases the anomalous interest takes its rise from the particular circumstances under which the instinct is pursued. The impulse to earn one's living is instinctive in origin ; some men earn their living by farming, therefore any subject which can be connected profitably with farming comes to be included in the interest, e.g., the chemical composition of a certain manure.

Sometimes, however, the connection with an instinct is more remote, and the interest tends to be deficient ; or the connection may be altogether wanting. A boy in school doing Latin grammar rarely sees any connection between the declension of *melior* and anything else in the world. A schoolgirl, asked to calculate the number of pounds of potatoes grown in a ten-acre field, when one square rod yields half a hundredweight, may be pardoned for not seeing how arithmetic enters into any of her vital purposes. In each of these cases, if we get attention at all, it is due to a special effort on the part of the person attending. Such attention is called *voluntary*, to distinguish it from the spontaneous attention that we give to objects that are really interesting. In ourselves we may frequently watch a conflict between the two types of attention. We are at the moment, say, writing an essay, and later are going to a dance. For us the dance is infinitely more interesting than the essay on " The Causes of the Franco-Prussian War ", but we are making an effort to attend to the latter. In spite of all we can do, thoughts of the dance keep slipping in between sentences on Bismarck or the unification of Germany, and we can only banish them as the result of repeated efforts at " concentration ". At the end, when we finish our essay, we are thoroughly tired.

To children, voluntary attention is probably even more fatiguing than it is to adults. A student knows more or less clearly the part that an essay on " The Franco-Prussian War " plays in his general scheme of things ; he wishes to earn his living by teaching, and essays are a step in the path towards the certificate necessary for teaching. If under these circumstances Bismarck still remains uninteresting to a comparatively mature student, it is small wonder that a child cannot bring his attention to bear steadily on Latin declensions or the output of potatoes.

If we expect children to give spontaneous attention to the tasks that they are set, we must manage to connect these tasks, either directly or indirectly, with the children's natural interests. In many cases this is simple. A child's instinctive interest in himself and his fellow-men rapidly expands to take in his district, country, or the history of mankind in different periods or districts. For this reason the human side of history and geography is receiving ever greater emphasis in teaching. Natural gregariousness expands to take in the organized group, and hence politics and the various forms of social organization become interesting; while curiosity and the interest in the partially strange will develop into a scientific attention to the surrounding world.

Many children are also captivated by the idea of doing " grown-up " things ; this motive helps them to realize the ultimate value of tasks they are set.

Some children of nine or ten years old willingly learn to sew or cook or look after a baby (instinctive interests play a part here), and almost any child in the top form of an elementary school will be interested in learning how to write a letter applying for a job. Personal ambition also may make otherwise dull facts interesting, as in the case of children who diligently work at uninteresting subjects in order to get a scholarship.

In some cases all these stimuli to interest are lacking, but attention is still possible—the attention, that is, which is purely voluntary. As we have said, this attention is unstable and fatiguing, and it is achieved by an effort of will. For this reason, as we have said above, it is often treated with extreme respect by educationists.

There is no doubt that it is of the greatest advantage to any man to have full voluntary control of his attention, so as to be able to attend to now this, and now that, as occasion demands, without being disturbed by irrelevant thoughts— but this power is not necessarily cultivated by attending to uninteresting matter. The safest course is to attempt to provide the child with the maximum number of interests, so that, for him, the number of uninteresting tasks in the world may be diminished, and effective attention be as easy as possible. The good work in business or elsewhere is not done by those who resolutely command an unruly train of thoughts, but by those who take an interest in their work and think about it without effort. Moreover, except to the stupid, few tasks are totally devoid of interesting features. We need to send our children out from school not with the expectation of being bored, but rather on the outlook for something to be interested in. If in school they have learnt to work for distant aims, and are accustomed to connect a present task with future achievement, they are better fitted to find interest in work which otherwise might be boring.

It is a fortunate dispensation of providence that voluntary attention to a certain subject generally ends by breeding spontaneous attention and interest. The cause is probably twofold. Progress in a subject reveals unexpected mines of wealth, and, as time goes on, we incorporate that subject into our self-regarding sentiment. A boy learning Latin passes from sentences such as *Pueri amant reginam* to the unexpected stories of Roman heroes, and then, maybe, to the epic of Hannibal. These topics appeal to natural interests, and Latin becomes a new source of gratification. Also the boy begins to think of himself as knowing Latin, takes a pride in his progress, and regards his knowledge as an accomplishment which his family and friends expect of him. Therefore, for his own honour he must do well in it. Thus voluntary attention is strengthened, to pass gradually into spontaneous interest as the subject opens out to him, and as efficiency in the subject becomes more and more necessary for the boy's own self-esteem.

Although the greater bulk of a person's interests can generally, with a little ingenuity, be explained as derived, directly or indirectly, from instincts, it is often hard to account for certain particular interests, or for the choice of one out of many possibilities. These particular interests are often determined early, apparently by chance, yet the same combination of circumstances would not have had the same effect on a different character. One enthusiastic mountaineer declared that his interest had started at the age of seven, when he had somehow found and read Tyndall's *Glaciers of the Alps*. One of the navy's most expert divers had formed a desire to enter that branch of the service from the time when he read one of the paper-backed novels, dear to boyhood, of adventures under sea. The present writer's introduction to psychology took place at thirteen, when she read Dr. C. S. Myers' *Experimental Psychology*, and thought it the most interesting book ever written. In others, who are generally called geniuses, these interests declare themselves earlier and with even less provocation. Schubert could write tunes at the age of seven, and the child Mozart, at five, was showing remarkable musical powers. Other children develop an extraordinary interest and ability in manipulating figures. There are many stories of " calculating boys ", but quite an ordinary child who possesses " a gift for figures " will show an astonishing knowledge of, and interest in, figures. A boy of this sort, aged 9½, knew all the numbers which were cubes or squares or multiples of interesting numbers (such as 13 or 17) up to three or four hundred. He was being given a lesson on decimals, and, although the connection with fractions had not been pointed out; he seemed to divine it, and promptly remarked, " I think we will have a sum with ·75 in it, because that is ¾, and I like working with ¾'s."

Such interests as these are generally connected with abilities. We like those subjects for which we have an aptitude. But the converse is also generally true—that if we can take an interest in a subject we shall do well at it. This connection is, however, by no means invariable. We fairly often see people with a real interest in a subject for which they have no aptitude, and more rarely we find that a person has ability for a subject which he dislikes, or at least is quite uninterested in. It is generally possible to trace this disinclination to some special circumstance.

If this is the origin of attention, what are its effects on mental processes ? From the care devoted to attaining it in schools these might be assumed to be something very important, and yet attention is frequently spoken of as if it were merely the reinforcement of one item of consciousness to the exclusion of all others from the mind. This is true as far as it goes, since if we attend closely to one thing, we are unaware of much that goes on around us. If we sit reading in a room which contains a loudly ticking clock, as long as we are enthralled by the book and attend closely to it, we do not notice the clock ; if we lay our book down, the ticking after a time catches our ear and gradually grows louder till the sound dominates our consciousness. There are many stories told of the absorption of eminent scientists in their work : they could suffer severe burns in the course of their experiments and not notice them ; and it is a well-known fact that most artists' wives have to summon their husbands to dinner. But attention is much more than this exclusion of all else in favour of a single idea or experience. The favoured idea is not *passively* received, but rather is dealt with actively by the mind. This active process is what gives attention its educational importance. If we attend to a lesson on Wales we do not simply hear the voice of the teacher, but we actively interweave what she says with our previous knowledge. We are always anticipating her statements, wondering if she will mention the mountains or towns that we know, correcting or amplifying our ideas about places, or seeing if we can recapitulate the information that has been given. We form associations between the new and the old and organize the new matter itself into a whole. It is just such organization and association that are the greatest aids to memory. Only in a wide sense is this attention unifocal (directed to a single object). We attend to the geography of Wales as a whole rather than to some single point in the lesson. If our attention were too closely focussed on one single idea, there could not be the association of different ideas which is so important an aspect of attention.

A consideration of what was said about the instinctive origin of attention will make this clear. Attention is essentially the precursor of action, and is part of the direction of a creature's activities to a certain end. In consequence, attention should not end with perception, e.g., the cat's perception of the scratch of a mouse is only the beginning of a full act of attention. Attention to the noise starts off the active process which leads to catching the mouse. As soon as the scratch is heard, it must be interpreted, the cat must connect the present situation with others in the past, and must devise means of catching this particular mouse. Moreover, the situation as a whole must be attended to—it would be useless if the animal became so absorbed in the pursuit of game that it itself became the prey of some larger creature. Nor must it attend too exclusively to some one aspect of the situation, so that it spends hours watching one mouse hole while the mouse escapes by another.[1]

Primitive attention is thus both purposive and comparatively dispersed. Man, living under rather different conditions, has, in many cases, developed a type of attention which is more restricted and more intense. We can see both types of attention still among civilized men. Some people will become absorbed in an idea or a task to such an extent that they are unable to give a thought to anything outside it : they forget to answer letters, miss their trains, or neglect their friends when any especially absorbing occupation arises. Others are unable to attend to any one thing for very long, and work best and most productively if they have continual change of occupation, and divide their periods of work by short spells of idleness. Each person who gives the matter any consideration can easily discover to which type he belongs, and should arrange his methods of work to suit his own type of mind.

The possibility of doing *two* things at once depends on one thing being more or less automatic. Any action which is quite habitual leaves the attention free for thought on some other subject. One can walk and argue with a friend ; and the process of brushing one's hair is often conducive to thought. The normal adult performs the mechanical parts of writing without any attention, and thus can pursue a train of thought without being in any way disturbed by the process of writing it down. If that same person tries to use a typewriter, an instrument in the use of which he is not skilled, he finds that thought is impossible, since all his efforts are concentrated on finding the keys ; yet the experi-

[1] A good example of the result of this dispersed attention has been given in the chapter on will.

enced typist finds the use of the machine no more disturbing to thought than the other finds a pen. Little children in schools are rather in the position of the amateur typist. Writing in itself presents so many difficulties that it often engrosses their whole attention and renders them incapable of doing any thinking if they are to write their best at the same time. Hence the failure of many young elementary school children in composition. Teachers kill children's ideas by an excessive emphasis on neatness in writing.

FOR DISCUSSION

1.—Make a list of your most prominent interests and try to show how they have been formed.

2.—Sketch the traditional methods of developing children's powers of attention used in schools and say how far you think them psychologically satisfactory.

3.—From a popular daily or weekly paper make a list of the topics which seem (from the size of the headline and amount of space allowed) to be most interesting to the mass of readers. Can you account for these interests by reference to instincts or to useful purposes ?

4.—Have you found it difficult or easy to attend to this chapter in this book ? What motives or methods have you used to hold your attention to the subject ?

5.—Mention some topics or sections of subjects which children usually find dull, but which are necessarily taught in schools. Suggest how you could present them so as to win voluntary attention from the class.

6.—Do you think it true that many interests may lead to dissipation of energy ? Consider cases of men who have had wide interests and yet have achieved much in any single branch of thought.

BOOKS

GEORGE H. GREEN, *Psycho-Analysis in the Class Room.* Especially Ch. vii. This discusses the nature and origin of interests.

DAY, *Sandford and Merton.* A novel dealing with a past form of education. It shows how a tutor attempts to rouse and satisfy two boys' interests.

RICHARD JEFFERIES, *Bevis, a Boy.* A children's book dealing with all sorts of things interesting to boys.

CHAPTER XIV

MEMORY

" I have forgot."
" Think well, there be means to make you remember."

IF the term memory be taken in its widest sense, its importance for mental life cannot be over-estimated, since it is the condition of all progress. In its widest sense memory means the conservation of experience so that the past affects action in the present. Without this conservation of experience we could not develop. If every time we repeated an action we did it no more skilfully than before, we should never achieve anything ; we should grow stronger than a baby, but no wiser. Thus memory operates both physically and mentally. By its aid we learn to use our limbs and adjust our movements ; to perceive objects in the world about us ; we come to understand " that the more one sickens the worse at ease he is . . . that the property of rain is to wet, and fire to burn ; that good pasture makes fat sheep, and that a great cause of the night is the lack of the sun " ; and we also acquire the more recondite knowledge " that he that hath learned no wit by nature, nor art, may complain of good breeding, or comes of a very dull kindred ".[1]

This general form of memory operates everywhere, and is so general that it can hardly receive special education. It improves with experience. From it arises the resourcefulness of the much-travelled man. To one who has had many experiences, seen many ways of dealing with unexpected situations, a store of expedients suggest themselves in cases where another man, of narrow experience, stands

[1] *As You Like It*, Act III., Sc. 2.

helpless. It is also the cause of that quality which is called good breeding. It is possible to learn good manners to some extent, but situations will always occur for which we have not been specifically prepared. One who has grown up among the usages of good society has a store of reactions which will carry him through life successfully.

In neither of these cases is the memory on which action depends explicit, any more than it is when we use our own language or another with which we are very familiar ; yet, as we know our own tongue because we have learnt it and still remember it, so our conduct on different occasions depends on a memory of previous behaviour. We realize the nature of this memory when anything disturbs its normal functioning. In fatigue many people find that they suffer from aphasia (that is, they cannot find the words that they need to express their meaning). In its commonest form this aphasia means that names are forgotten, but it sometimes becomes so acute in certain pathological states that the patient cannot speak at all, or only a few disconnected words. A corresponding state in which a person lost the power to understand meanings was once reported to the writer. The patient heard a voice speaking but could no longer, without laborious effort, interpret the sounds as being words ; she had temporarily lost that part of her memory.

More usually the term memory is used in a limited sense, meaning that we remember something in particular, and do so with more or less of an effort. There are many stages between general recall, such as that discussed above, and memory for special things. There is much difference of effort between the easy speaking of one's own tongue and the agonized search for a name which eludes us. Yet in all cases the same mechanism is at work, the difference lying in the ease with which the memory works.

We can distinguish three aspects of an act of memory : the impression, the retention, and the reproduction. Obviously we must have perceived a thing before we can remember it, and some impression must be retained or it could not influence our conduct later. In a complete act of memory all three aspects are clear, but we often fail in the third, though the first and second parts are operative. In such a case we get recognition without full memory.   The most obvious case occurs when we wish to tell someone the name of the friend who enquired so tenderly after his welfare.   We rack our brain, fail to recollect it, and finally say, " Repeat the likely names and I'll tell you when you come to it."   We can recognize the name when it is said, though we cannot say it ourselves.   In a similar way there are a large number of things that we recognize though we should never think of trying to reproduce them.   There are many pictures that we know well, though we could hardly make even the roughest sketch of one from memory.   In an experiment to be mentioned later, the subject recognizes blots or geometrical figures which have been shown once, though probably he could not draw any of them.

There is no hard and fast line between mere recognition and full memory.   We can observe this if we read a piece of poetry several times and attempt to repeat it after each reading.   Our success increases gradually from the first time when we know the sense and a few words here and there, through all stages of completeness till, in the end, we are word-perfect.

For educational purposes it is expedient to make a division between two types of memory.   The distinction is due to Bergson [1] and has considerable importance.   Roughly, the distinction is as follows.   Much of the matter that we remember has been presented once or a few times only.   We remember at lunch the events of the morning just passed, and they occurred once only ; on the other hand, some of our memories have been acquired by dint of much repetition, as, for example, our knowledge of a certain poem.   These memories differ by more than their mode of origin ;   our memory of an interview may enable us to repeat the actual words of the conversation, but generally the meaning of the whole scene is retained rather than the exact details.   On the other hand, when we have learnt a poem, what we have achieved is a language *habit* of reciting the words.   We may, or we may not, know what the words mean, but we can remember and repeat the sounds in their correct order.   Our understanding of the matter may affect the rate of learning, but when once the words are learnt, we can remember them,

[1] Bergson, *Matter and Memory.*

whether they have meaning or whether they are to us merely senseless syllables. It is convenient to refer to these two types of memory as pure memory and habit memory. Bergson uses this distinction to throw light on the nature of the soul. We need not follow him into metaphysics, but we can use his distinction for guidance in education. Too often in the past education has relied almost exclusively on habit memory. Children have been asked to learn the dates of the kings of England, or the capes and bays of North America, merely by repetition, without any intelligent understanding of what they were doing ; or they learnt by heart Latin verse, which they probably could not translate. The method was one of repetition and testing ; of compiling lists and " getting them off ", and was, in essence, similar to that in use in the schools of the East, where the children chant over and over again the sacred books, until they can repeat them by rote.

The present tendency is away from habit learning. In learning by heart, and especially in learning facts, it is far quicker to employ pure memory, either wholly or in part, than to rely solely on habit memory. A few repetitions when accompanied by thorough understanding can take the place of much chanting or revision, and so the drudgery of wearisome unintelligent repetition is saved.

With this change in the method of learning goes a change in the type of material presented. Anything can be learnt by habit memory, if sufficient time is given to it, but for pure memory it is necessary that the matter presented should have *meaning*. For a lazy teacher the old style of teaching is easier, as he need make no effort to choose interesting material, nor need he bother to explain it. Now, if pure memory rather than habit memory is to be employed, the teacher must arrange the material so that it has the maximum meaning and interest for the class. If matter is to be memorized rapidly, it must not only possess meaning for the pupil, but it must also interest him. The stimulus of fear may keep children working at matter which is repeated again and again until it is known, but when uninteresting matter is presented once or twice only, the child will certainly never remember it. On the other hand, tell an interesting story once to a child and he will often remember it so accurately that he will correct you if you make any alterations when you tell it to him a second time.

The different school subjects vary in the opportunities they offer for using pure memory. In subjects like history and geography, though names and dates often have to be learnt by repetition, the bulk of the matter, if it is presented in the form of stories, or of facts clearly and logically interconnected, can be retained at once. In arithmetic, when the method of working a sum has been understood, no further mechanical repetition of principles is necessary, although practice may be necessary to give skill and accuracy. On the other hand, it is impossible to dispense with repetition in learning arithmetical tables. It is an excellent thing to show children how the tables are built up, but when they are doing sums they are handicapped if they are not perfectly familiar with their tables.

In languages, too, a large part of the work must be done by habit memory. One can understand the rules of grammar and syntax, but nothing but repetition will fix a vocabulary in one's memory. Yet the use of the vocabulary can be made intelligent. The " direct " method leads the child to use the new words in an interesting way, whereas under the older methods the pupil learnt lists of unrelated words. In learning poetry, both forms of memory naturally co-operate.

As both forms of memory must be used in schools it is well to consider the conditions most favourable to the working of each.

1. HABIT MEMORY

(a) This depends essentially on repetition, and if this repetition can be done rhythmically, so much the better. Some children learn their multiplication tables to a march tune, and this is probably helpful. Much matter is presented in metrical form for this reason. We all know the days in each month from a rhyme, and every schoolboy who learns Latin knows that :

> a, ab, absque, coram, de,
> palam, clam, cum, ex and e,

take the ablative, and remembers the fact all the better because of the swing of the lines. For the same reason, too, it is easier to learn verse by heart than it is to learn prose, and, though it may be good for children in school to learn noble prose, it will take a longer time, and they will forget it more rapidly, than they would a piece of verse of corresponding length. This accounts for the early metrical versions of stories, rules and laws, counsel and facts. Rhyme and rhythm fix the words in the mind, so that ballads, runes, psalms, and the " few rhymed precepts " to be carried in the memory are amongst the older forms of literature.

(*b*) An important part is played in learning by attempted reproduction. A child is anxious to say his poem to the teacher long before he really knows it. This is irritating for the teacher of a large class, but it is the outcome of a real need in the child. The effort of reproduction impresses those parts which the child knows and he sees clearly just where his knowledge fails, and so is able to supplement his special deficiencies. Experiments have shown that a high proportion of attempted reproduction to repetition from the book gives the most rapid memorizing.

(*c*) The method of presenting the material to be learnt is also important. Some people learn best if they can see the words, for they remember " where so-and-so comes on the page " ; some wish to hear the piece ; others require to pronounce the words themselves. In consequence, with a class of children the ideal is to present the matter in all three ways and then each child will get that most suitable to himself. If the children have copies of the poem to be learnt, hear it well read by the teacher, and are allowed to say it to themselves, all methods are brought into use. Often children are wiser than their teacher and start murmuring over what they are required to learn. Some teachers stop this. Of course, it must be stopped if the noise is loud enough to disturb other classes, but if it is not, the children's practice is psychologically the right one.

Each child should be encouraged to discover for himself which method, or combination of methods, is best for him, and he should use that method, for no two people have exactly the same ways of doing anything, and in mental work there is no " one best way ".

(*d*) In all learning it is most important to avoid fatigue, as matter learnt when we are tired is very rapidly forgotten. Lessons involving learning by heart should be put at times when the class is reasonably fresh. These lessons should not be very long. It is more economical to work at learning something for two periods of fifteen minutes each, than for one of thirty minutes. It is more advantageous to have five spelling lessons of ten minutes each in the week than one of fifty, and it is better to work at tables for three minutes at the beginning and end of each arithmetic lesson in the week, than for fifteen minutes all at once. This fact has been well established by experiment, and it is possible to test it personally if one is engaged in learning a foreign language. A weekly coaching gives most disappointing results. It is only if one devotes a certain amount of time to the subject every day that any real progress becomes apparent.

(e) For permanent retention spaced revision is necessary. If a poem is learnt on Monday the most effective arrangement of revision which is intended to give permanent retention, is something as follows : The poem might be revised on Tuesday (when owing to a curious phenomenon called reminiscence it might be better known than it was on Monday), on Thursday, on the following Monday, and perhaps in another week's time. The revision should be divided by longer and longer periods as time goes on, and be most frequent immediately after the first learning. The reason for this is that obliviscence is most rapid just after the matter has been learnt, but what has been retained after the first day or two is forgotten slowly. Revision is obviously most necessary when the rate of forgetting is highest.

(f) Lastly, and this as well as (d) applies to all types of memory, it is more economical to learn in wholes than in parts. In learning a poem of moderate length it is a better practice to read it right through several times than to read two or three lines or a single verse and repeat that part until it is known, and then go on to another part, and so on. The reason for this is that the poem makes less sense when taken in fragments, and, therefore, pure memory is less active. Also wrong associations are formed between the end and beginning of the same section, instead of the correct association between the end of one section and the beginning of the succeeding one.

In consequence, a lesson of the following type is psychologically indefensible, yet it can be heard in almost any school. The time is 3.30 p.m., the class is sleepy, and so perhaps is the teacher. The time-table says " Recitation ", and the lesson is proceeding as follows : " All sit still, fold your arms, shut your lips. Now we are going to learn a hymn. I will read it out to you and you shall say it after me." The teacher begins to intone : " ' Now the day is over.' Now say that." The class does so. The teacher continues : " Night is drawing nigh." At the end of the verse the teacher says : " Now say the whole verse." There is complete failure ; yet the lesson continues in the same manner till the bell gives release at four o'clock. The impressions in children's minds which result from such methods of learning are amazing. Those of us who learnt the Commandments or Catechism in the days of our extreme youth, can provide many examples of this. One child was accustomed to say, when reciting the Lord's Prayer, " Alice will be my name," instead of " hallowed be Thy Name ", and was never troubled by the thought of this strange provision for the future.

2. PURE MEMORY

This is influenced to a far greater extent by the subject matter than habit memory is, and it can be affected by the method of learning in the same way.

(a) If we contrast the ease with which we learn such a sentence as " THE FAT CAT IS WELL " with the number of repetitions required to learn a list of nonsense syllables such as NUF, SAS, BAC, DEP, YOT, although there are the same number of syllables in each case, we have a rough measure of the importance of *meaning* in aiding memory.

In regard to meaning there are two main points to be considered when teaching : (1) is the matter to be learnt sufficiently within the children's experience to be emotionally comprehensible ? and (2) is it conveyed in language which is within their understanding ? In the first case, much that would of itself be incomprehensible to little children (e.g., life in distant lands) may be made comprehensible, in some degree, by being connected with their actual experience. It is easier to understand the Sahara if one knows sand hills at home, or arctic life if one is well acquainted with snow. Yet, even with this help, much must remain incomprehensible to children and had better be omitted. It is useless to attempt to teach small children poetry which concerns adult passions of love or longing, unless these passions are reduced to simple child-like dimensions, as are the love-affairs of the prince and princess of fairy-tales.

In regard to the language much can be done by anticipating the children's difficulties and explaining them in advance. This is preferable to reading the passage, or giving the lesson, and then asking if the children have understood, or questioning them on difficult points to convict them of ignorance. A previous explanation aids understanding and, therefore, aids memory, and also gives the child the pleasure of recognition when he hears the point touched on in the lesson itself. This does not mean that the children shall not be made to think, since, even in a previous explanation, use can be made of the context, or of the etymology of the words or phrases, to help the children to arrive at the meaning for themselves.

If, in spite of the teacher's care, a phrase or a fact remains which the children do not understand, it is almost certain to be mis-remembered. In a certain memory test given to girls of 14 the phrase " patron of art " occurred. The experimenters had not imagined that this would cause any difficulty, but a large proportion of the children left it out when reproducing the story, while many others turned it into " a master of arts ". As these children lived in Cambridge they were obviously substituting a familiar for an unknown phrase.

(b) Pure memory is also to a large extent dependent on association. The more associations that are formed between one fact and others, the more easily will that fact be recalled. These associations may either be between old matter and a new fact, or between a number of new facts. In the former case the term generally used is " apperception ", a term invented by the German educationist, Herbart, to describe the process by which a new fact is absorbed into a body of existing knowledge. Suppose we are well acquainted with the facts of Edmund Spenser's life and with his poems, and are then told that a parody of the first lines of the *Faery Queene* occurs in a play called the *Return from Parnassus*, acted about 1601 ; we may easily remember this new fact, for it is associated with other ideas in which we are or have been interested ; but if, being ignorant of astronomy, we are told that a certain star is not a unity, as it appears, but a group of four, the chances are that we shall forget the name of the star at once. In the former case there was a body of knowledge to which the new fact adhered ; in the second, the fact was isolated and consequently soon lost. In teaching it is necessary to keep this in mind. We must try to lead up to new knowledge from that which the children already possess. In consequence, the beginning of many lessons should be devoted to seeing that the children have in their minds a suitable body of ideas ready to receive the new facts which will be given them. Thus it is a good thing to start a lesson on the Elizabethan seamen by a few revision questions on the position and discovery of the New World, but such questions would be worse than useless if the lesson to follow were on the social troubles of Richard II's reign. The *indiscriminate* " revision of the last lesson ", which occurs in so many lesson notes, is a psychologically disadvantageous practice.

Within the lesson itself much can be done to aid the memory by showing the connexion between the different new facts presented. We want our lesson to be a connected whole, not a number of isolated facts, however interesting these may be in themselves. As an extreme example, take the performance at a party of the witty man who tells one funny story after another. The listeners laugh and enjoy it thoroughly, yet, at the end, few could repeat any of the jokes that were not already familiar. The same audience, however, could remember the larger part of a well-arranged lecture, even though they were not particularly interested in it at the time.

One of the best methods for ensuring association of newly learnt knowledge is to use it. The use should not be mere reproduction of the lesson given ; it should also involve old knowledge and an extension beyond the particular matter taught. The children, moreover, should have to employ some personal originality and effort in using the new knowledge gained. Thus, after a lesson on the climatic conditions of England, the children could use the knowledge so gained to predict the climate of some other region not yet studied. The importance of this use of knowledge has led to the catch phrase in education " no impression without expression ", which means simply that we don't know a thing properly till we have used our knowledge.

(c) The third most important factor in determining memory is interest. In the last chapter the effect of interest on attention was discussed and the way in which attention assisted in the organization of one fact with another. The value of this for memory is obvious from what has been said above, and we can, from our own experience, see how much our memory is affected by our interests. If we are followers of the league matches, we know the names of the teams, the divisions in which they play, and the chances each has of the cup. If we are uninterested, all this information slips out of our mind the minute it enters it. The same is true of school subjects. One child has a good memory for history but can't remember geography, though the subject matter is not very different—at least, as often taught in schools. From the things that people remember it is often possible to deduce their interests. An amusing experiment is to get a number of people to read the same book of short stories, and then, after an interval, to ask each person which story he remembers best. Many curious conclusions may be based on the answers.

The distinction between pure and habit memory has been made for convenience of exposition. It must not be imagined that either works, or should work, separately. It is all to the good that both should be employed over any piece of learning, only the *proportion* of each used in any piece of mental work differs. Very few people can learn anything accurately at a single presentation ; a second or third reading is necessary before the matter is fixed in the mind. On the other hand, it is extremely risky, besides being laborious, to employ habit memory alone. Pure memory, with its grasp of principles and meaning, supplies an invaluable check on the common inaccuracies of habit memory. Speaking generally, we may say that the more stupid a student is, the more he employs habit memory, the slower he works, and the more inaccurate his memory is. The nonsensical misquotations, which disfigure many English papers, are evidences of this. The students, who in a recent examination wrote : " The *steering* spires of Oxford," or " Playing the *credulous* ape to Shakespeare," had attempted to remember the words without any regard for the sense. As a matter of policy, both in learning and teaching, the best plan is to go first for the sense of anything to be learnt, and then, when that is clear, to learn by heart such details or quotations as are seen to be important from this point of view.

In acts of memory we can generally observe the same purposive character which characterizes other mental acts. This is especially noticeable with pure memory. Habit memory, like any other habit, will retain any action which it is required to retain, and is in the nature of a *tool* rather than of a directing power of mind ; but pure memory, working by meaning and selectively, is—as we shall show presently—well adapted for carrying out purposes. In most cases, it is the meaning of a situation or the sense of a book that is important for subsequent action. The details may also be important, as in a book on engineering, but even there the main value lies in the general principles. So too, in active life, when we recall an interview, it is what the people *meant* which matters most for our subsequent conduct.[1] Pure memory seizes on these meanings, and it is characteristic of it to retain them rather than particular details. Furthermore, we do not as a rule remember a complete scene. We only remember part, and this part will generally be relevant to our purposes at the moment of recollection. If we have been on a walking tour and are describing it to a botanist, we try to give an account of the flowers we found, and, at the time of speaking, we remember these more vividly than anything else. When later we talk to an artist we are full of information about colour effects of

[1] Unless of course we are seeking evidence for a lawsuit.

sea and early budding trees. On the whole it is a mark of low intellectual ability to remember in too great detail when that detail is not relative to the matter in hand.

This account presupposes that different parts of our total memories are available at different times, and this presupposition is certainly true. In all honesty one may be ignorant of a fact one minute and recall it shortly after. These memories are sometimes recoverable by a trick, sometimes they return spontaneously in moments of reverie, or just before falling asleep. It is wrong, therefore, to accuse a child of lying or carelessness if he asserts that he does not know something which we have every reason to believe that he does know.

Apart from memories which are temporarily inaccessible, there are others which are accessible, but are so faint at the time that they are passed over as if forgotten. Yet they will return when circumstances call for them. Frequently one can only remember names of places when in the particular district to which these names belong. A child who spends his Easter holidays in Wales and his summer ones in Cornwall may be unable to recollect the names of either set of familiar places when back in London for term time, yet each set returns in the proper locality.

An even more remarkable example of the purposiveness of memory is the way relevant facts suggest themselves in the course of work. The examples contained in this book were almost all recalled *ad hoc* as the pages were written, though many of them are incidents which occurred years ago. The right examples suggested themselves for each chapter, and probably no amount of previous thinking would have caused them to occur to the mind.

Not only remembering is purposive, so also is forgetting. The extreme form of this doctrine, as put forward by Freud, has caused much misunderstanding and much annoyance, but the general statement is true. In the first place, given memory, forgetting is a necessary function. If we retained every impression, fresh and vivid, our minds would resemble nothing so much as an over-crowded museum, and any real thought would be impossible. We must forget, either temporarily or permanently, if there is to be any order and emphasis in our thoughts. We therefore forget the unimportant, our past college meals, the numbers of our rooms at hotels, the bills we have paid and put on the receipt file. Sometimes, something of importance gets forgotten, too, among the other lumber, but that is generally because we only learnt its value too late.

The purposive nature of our forgetting, however, goes beyond this. We forget much that we do not *want* to remember, not just those things we do not *need* to remember. The rapidity with which we forget the exact sensations of a pain has often been commented on. Sea-sickness may overwhelm us for hours, yet within half an hour of landing may be almost forgotten.

There are, too, a number of slightly unpleasant things which are constantly " slipping our mind ". Engagements with the dentist, invitations to tea with people who bore us, income tax schedules to be filled up, or the order to the grocer which we have been commissioned to give.

In certain cases, bordering on the pathological, more important things are forgotten ; and, if we investigate, we shall generally find that the event forgotten was unpleasant. In the same way, nightmares are often forgotten by the dreamer, though the person to whom they were told remembers them well. Lastly, in cases of shell-shock during the War, large parts of the patients' experience were forgotten. The task of the physician was to bring back these forgotten incidents to the conscious memory of the patient, and to help him to face their unpleasantness in a rational way.

What then is a good memory ? One that learns readily, retains important things permanently, and keeps them readily accessible for the needs of the moment ; since it is no good knowing a great many things if we cannot produce the particular piece of information required at the right time.

There are great differences in individual endowment in memory. Some people have a very good habit memory, and can learn names and figures rapidly and retain them well ; others may learn languages badly, yet be good at any subject which involves more pure memory. Others again are blessed with both types. There are also differences in such qualities as the accuracy with which things are recalled, or the type of matter most easily remembered. Certain people have wonderful memories for figures, while others can recall names and faces in a way that appears marvellous to those not similarly gifted. Again, nearly everyone can remember well in the line of his special interests, but some people can remember anything that comes along. Such people become encyclopædias as the years go by, and if they are dull men, become the most unconscionable bores ; but if brilliant, the best talkers in the world.

Many psychological quacks offer to improve the memory for modest sums of £3 3s., or so. The possibility of their really doing this is small. It is quite easy to improve the technique of memory and thus to improve the amount memorized. It is also possible to increase one's circle of interests, and, as memory follows interest, this serves to increase the number of things remembered ; but native endowment of memory seems little capable of direct improvement, although, up to a point, memory develops with age. The power to learn increases up to about the age of 25, the power to retain what is learnt up to about the age of 12 ; so that though it is not true to say that children learn more quickly than adults, it is true to say that what is learnt in childhood is retained better than material learnt later. In extreme old age the power to retain new impressions is sometimes lost entirely, though the events of youth are still clearly in mind.

As knowledge becomes more voluminous, the importance of memory decreases. Nowadays, it is more important to know where to find information than to have it actually in mind at the moment. The same thing is happening in business ; elaborate systems of indexing are replacing the old method of keeping a fact in one's head, and though memory is still of great importance, it is receiving so much assistance from other sources that its training is no longer the vital matter it once was.

Lastly, what is the justice of the charge that too much attention to memory is deleterious to originality ? We cannot have serviceable originality unless it is based on the accumulated knowledge of the race and, therefore, on memory, but the two must be combined. The learning of facts for their own sake is deadening. Facts should be learnt for use and recombined to meet ever new problems.

In this way invention and originality are stimulated, and the knowledge possessed by the individual becomes mobile and so readily available.

FOR DISCUSSION

1.—Account for the fact that an actor finds it increasingly easy to learn new parts by heart.
2.—What were the theories by which educators of a generation ago justified the learning by heart of 500 lines of poetry, e.g., " The Deserted Village," with little reference to appreciation or understanding ? Refute the theories if you can.
3.—Describe clearly your own methods of learning :
   (a) A sonnet.
   (b) A longer poem, e.g., " The Ode on the Death of the Duke of Wellington."
   (c) The parts of a Latin or French verb.
   (d) A drill " Table ".
   (e) An address or a telephone number.
4.—Describe, from your own experience, instances where you have not been able to remember a name or a fact at the time you wanted it, but have suddenly remembered it later.
5.—What justification is there for letting children learn a passage by heart which they cannot at the time entirely understand.
6.—Procure, if you can, the prospectus of a " Mind-Training " Institution, and discover what methods are used there to " train " memory.
7.—What place is there in History, Geography and Scripture for the use of habit memory ?
8.—Discuss the advisability of getting into the way of " writing everything down ".
9.—Name any famous people you know who have been remarkable for encyclopædic or abnormally retentive memories, and show to what use they have put this gift.
10.—Suppose you have naturally a poor memory for faces and names. How could you help yourself to learn quickly the names of the children in your class ?

BOOKS

John Adams, *Herbartian Psychology.* Ch. iii. contains an account of Herbart's psychology and of apperception.
Pear, *Remembering and Forgetting.* Gives an account of the modern theories of memory, and explains why we forget.
Rusk, *Experimental Education.* This book contains accounts, among others, of the type of experiment on memory that is performed in schools.
F. Watt, *Economy and Training of Memory.* This is a little book full of practical hints about memory.
T. P. Nunn, *Education, Its Data and First Principles.* Especially important for the discussion of memory (called " mneme ") under its widest aspect.

CHAPTER XV

IMAGERY AND IMAGINATION

" Good Sir, whose powers are these ? . . . and who commands them ? "

THE nature of imagination is somewhat difficult to understand, chiefly because of the ambiguity of the word as commonly used. This ambiguity attaches mainly to the verb imagine, which is used in two senses which are really distinct ; in one case it corresponds to the noun imagination, in the other to the noun image, and in psychology the two words have a very different meaning. We say we have a mental image when, without there being any external object to initiate the sensation, we have a mental experience such as might be given through any sense organ. Thus, as we dress in our bedroom, we can have an image of our breakfast table and see the food, the flowers and other appurtenances with more or less clearness ; we can hear over again, i.e., have an auditory image of the " Gilbert and Sullivan " we heard last week, or we can see and feel, as images, the movements necessary for cutting a figure 8 in skating. We can also have images of taste and smell, though many people have these images less readily than visual or auditory ones.

Also, with most images, we can feel with varying strength the emotion which would accompany such images if the things they represent were really present. When we image a lemon, our mouths water ; when we image a gay tune, we feel cheered ; when the image of a dead friend flashes into our mind, we feel a pang of sorrow akin to that felt when we first suffered loss. When the lover thinks of his beloved, his pulse quickens and he smiles with pleasure. In ordinary speech we say we " imagine " such images as these. In more correct psychological terminology we should say we " image " them ; thus reserving " imagine " for a rather different process. *Imagination* means more than these images, it indicates that something *new* is evolved. We will discuss this later.

If we make here a distinction for convenience it does not mean that the two processes are divided by a sharp line. Images are an essential part of imagination, and no one can say, or have any real reason for trying to say, where mere imagery ends and imagination begins. As will be said later, much of the distinction between the two processes depends on a judgment of value, and if we are to avoid cant in education it is important to make up our minds to what processes the different words we use refer ; so that we shall not say that we are " cultivating imagination " when we are only encouraging imagery, or condemn day-dreaming (which is a kind of imagination) while labouring to produce something which we call by a different name, but which is in fact almost exactly the same thing.

Images fall into two classes : there are those which concern the past and are more or less faithful reproductions of past events, and there are those which concern the future or the unexperienced. The former are not imagination, the latter generally are. If we look back on a holiday, certain events stand out in our memory, pictures rise in our mind of cliffs and sea, we feel the warm wind and smell the gorse and the salt in the air, and we experience the sweet content of pleasant companionship. These are memory images, and they are of different vividness in different people. In some they are faint, in others they are strong and accompanied by great pleasure.

> And oft when on my couch I lie
> In vacant or in pensive mood,
> They flash across that inward eye
> Which is the bliss of solitude,
> And then my heart with pleasure fills
> And dances with the daffodils.[1]

There is no doubt that such memory images add greatly to the enjoyment of life, and moreover they serve a useful

[1] Wordsworth, *The Daffodils.*

purpose in thought. Often the past is a guide to the future, and to be able to revive the past may be a great assistance in directing our present behaviour. Suppose we have been for a walk along a certain road and are then, some days later, asked to help a friend to drive his motor-car along that same road in the dark. At each corner we try to summon up an image of the turning as we saw it by daylight, so as to be able to say whether it is a sharp turn, whether a duck pond lies dangerously near the edge of the road, or whether there is a second bend just beyond the first. Images may rise very slowly and reluctantly and the whole experience may be one of painful effort. On the other hand, memory images often spring up unbidden to guide our action. When carrying a tray down a dark flight of stairs we may suddenly have an image of a box which we left standing at the bottom, and which we should trip over if we did not keep well away to the right-hand side.

There seems every probability that this type of memory image is very old. Before language was invented, the past experience of each man must have been retained—so far as it was retained—as a series of images. Early " picture-writing " testifies to this method of recording experience by images. It took many centuries for the pictures to become conventionalized into the symbols of linear writing.

Nearly as primitive must have been the use of images for prospective thinking. We try out a great many of our future actions in images before we actually do them. If we are going to make a table or stool in wood, we image it and consider the advantages and disadvantages of each type of construction before we actually begin. If we are careful, we test our image as far as possible by making a drawing before we start on our wood, and only then do we put our plan into practice.

Here again there are wide individual differences. Some people have wonderful control of their images. They can image clearly a bottle, pour out a glass of red wine from it, hold up the glass and watch the light in it—all in images. Others only construct images with great trouble and then the images are faint. A certain number of professions must depend very largely on this power to image. A producer of plays, or a designer of scenarios, must have control of his imagery and it must be vivid. It is of the greatest advantage to a novelist to have good powers of imagery. Anthony Trollope in his autobiography writes :

" The novelist has other aims than the elucidation of his plot. He desires to make his readers so intimately acquainted with his characters that the creatures of his brain should be to them speaking, moving, living, human creatures. This he can never do unless he knows these personages of fiction himself, and he can never know them unless he can live with them in the full reality of established intimacy. . . . I have so lived with my characters and thence has come whatever success I have obtained. There is a gallery of them, and in that gallery I may say that I know the tone of the voice, and the colour of the hair, every flame of the eye and the very clothes they wear."

Thackeray tells how a certain Costigan, a character in *Pendennis* whom he had invented some ten years earlier, once met him. " I was smoking in a tavern parlour one night and this Costigan came into the room alive, the very man : the most remarkable resemblance of the printed sketches of the man, of the rude drawings in which I had depicted him. He had the same little coat, the same battered hat cocked on one eye, the same twinkle in that eye. ' Sir,' said I, knowing him to be an old friend whom I had met in unknown regions, ' Sir,' I said, ' may I offer you a glass of brandy and water ? ' ' Bedad, ye may,' says he, ' and I'll sing ye a song tu.' Of course, he spoke with an Irish brogue. Of course, he had been in the army. . . ."

The power thus to recognize a character shows in what a concrete fashion Thackeray had imaged him.

In schools this faculty of definite imagery may be useful to children in many ways. It is a great assistance in all forms of mental arithmetic, especially when this exercise involves more than the mere application of some quick formula. In the same way visual imagery is of great assistance in spelling, in which a poor visualizer is severely handicapped. For such out-of-school activities as dressmaking or designing, visual imagery is almost indispensable, and even in the appreciation of poetry the visualizer has an advantage. The work of some poets is so rich in imagery that a reader possessed of poor or unready imagery is almost unable to appreciate the pictures of the verse, especially when these pictures change as rapidly as they do in the works of Shelley or Browning. The cultivation of imagery in schools, therefore, is desirable, but it is a mistake to speak of this cultivation as a " training in imagination ".

There are, however, certain children who suffer rather than gain from too vivid imagery. In school the concrete nature of the imagery may intervene to prevent them using numbers in arithmetic as symbols, and later in life a dependence on visual imagery may make a study of philosophy or logic difficult. Out of school also the vivid visualizer suffers, and shadows, which to most children are harmless, for him assume the guise of monsters.

Imagination is more than prospective imagery ; it is the " creative faculty of the mind " as the dictionary says. This definition is not really complete, but it is hard to give one that is more so. The best *description* of imagination is contained in the speech of Duke Theseus in *Midsummer Night's Dream*, which begins :

> More strange than true : I never may believe
> These antique fables, nor these fairy toys.

and which continues—

> The poet's eye, in a fine frenzy rolling,
> Doth glance from heaven to earth, from earth to heaven ;
> And, as imagination bodies forth
> The forms of things unknown, the poet's pen
> Turns them to shapes, and gives to airy nothings
> A local habitation and a name.[1]

This description emphasizes the qualities of imagination which are really important—that it involves the creation of something new ; that in the process of this creation images play their part ; and that the final result takes on concrete form. From this account it is clear that the difference between imagination and prospective or constructive imagery is the comparative novelty of the thing imagined. We should hardly call an ordinary frock a work of imagination, yet the characters of the novelist, though they are often made up " out of scraps, heel-taps, odds and ends of

[1] *Midsummer Night's Dream*, Act v., Sc. 1.

characters " previously known, are generally rightly said to be imagined. Our dreams are strangely on the border-line. We do not generally call them works of imagination (though with many people they are often very good stories) [1] because we do not have any experience of personal creation, and we regard our imaginings as our own creation. Dreams are presented to us in so matter of fact a way that we hardly regard them as our invention any more than we claim the world around us as our own construction. When, however, we are conscious of setting our inventive powers to work, then we claim our subsequent experiences as imagination. The following account illustrates an imagining which was perhaps half a dream of fever.

" While waiting for midnight to strike, I said to myself, thinking of yesterday and to-morrow . . . ' Yesterday is now twenty-four hours away, but in a minute it will only be one minute away.' I treated the hidden to-morrow similarly. I imagined, the world being old and creaky, ill-fitting too, that a crack existed between the two days. Anyone who was thin enough might slip through! I certainly was thin enough. I slipped through . . . I entered a region out of time, a region where everything came true. And the first thing I saw was a wondrous streaming vision of the wind, the wind that howled outside my filthy windows . . . I *saw* the winds, changing colours as they rose and fell, attached to the trees, in tenuous ribands of gold and blue and scarlet as they swept to and fro. . . ." [2]

The general nature of imagination would have been fairly clear from such descriptions as this, if Wordsworth and others had not darkened counsel by attempting to give imagination (as distinguished from fancy) a mythical value, and if " practical " men had not disparaged one of the most important aspects of imagination by labelling it day-dreaming. Wordsworth, in his preface to the edition of 1815, [3] attempts to indicate the nature of imagination. His account is most confused—as well it might be when he was

---

[1] R. L. Stevenson used dreams as the basis of several of his stories, e.g., *Dr. Jekyll and Mr. Hyde.*
[2] A. Blackwood, *Episodes Before Thirty*, p. 123. (The whole book can be recommended.)
[3] Oxford ed., p. 954.

trying to find distinctions where none really exist—and the easiest method of arriving at any definite idea of his doctrine is to look at his own classification of poems into those of the Fancy and those of the Imagination. In the former class are poems to a *Daisy*, the *Small Celandine, On seeing a needlecase in the form of a harp*, and so on. Under the head of Imagination are classed *Yew Trees, Simplon Pass* and many others of his most famous poems. Arguing from this we can roughly say that Imagination is the power which sees connections and affinities which belong to the heart of things, whereas fancy plays with external similarities. The *Daisy* is :

> A little cyclops with one eye
> Staring to threaten and defy,
> That thought comes next—and instantly
> The freak is over,
> The shape will vanish, and behold
> A silver shield with boss of gold,
> That spreads itself, some faery bold
> In fight to cover.

These idle similes are very different in value from the imaginings which revealed to Wordsworth the mystical unity underlying diversity which he tells of in *Tintern Abbey* and other poems.[1]

Many people who advocate the cultivation of imagination condemn the day-dream. The day-dream is supposed not to lead to action and is, therefore, set aside as valueless. But, from the point of view of psychology, considerations of value do not alter the nature of the phenomenon, which is one and the same whether it is called fancy, imagination or day-dreaming.

Those who believe they possess it regard imagination as a gift of the highest importance. Their worst condemnation of a person they dislike is, " he has no imagination ". The excuse for this attitude is that certain forms of imagination are of the greatest social value.

(1) Imagination and sympathy are closely connected. Sympathy arises when the sympathizer and the sufferer are brought into close contact ; imagination may produce the

---

[1] V. for example, *The Prelude, Toussaint l'Ouverture*, " The world is too much with us ".

same result in cases where they never meet ; for, as was said earlier in this chapter, a vivid mental picture of a situation produces, in some degree, the same emotion which would accompany the situation if it were actually present. This imagery is of the greatest importance in social life. If we are able to anticipate the feeling of those about us we can arrange our behaviour so as to cause the greatest pleasure or the reverse. If we are insensitive or lack foresight, we may err simply through ignorance, and with no intent to wound. The tactless man is deficient in this power of emotional imagination ; so, frequently, is the stupid man : whereas there are certain people who possess this insight into other people's feelings to an uncanny extent. This power they can use for good or ill, and, just as they may be the most delightful companions or friends, so, if other characteristics intervene, they can be a terror to all who come into contact with them, especially their subordinates. Their refined power to wound keeps them from mere brutality, and leaves the victim more helpless than if he had a more specific injury.[1] The gift of imaginative sympathy is indispensable to the dramatist if his characters are to behave in a life-like and convincing way. Similarly in acting, the actor must imaginatively put himself in the place of the characters represented and live through their experiences—at least, to some extent. This is one of the ways in which drama is useful in schools. Acting forces children to make this effort at sympathetic imagination, and thus accustoms them, if only in a small degree, to think of the feelings of others placed in various circumstances.

This sympathetic imagination works only if we feel ourselves akin to the other party. The horrors of the slave trade, or the campaigns of extermination carried out in Elizabethan Ireland, or in more modern Tasmania, were tolerable only so long as no one concerned ever asked himself " How should *I* feel in similar circumstances ? " The sufferers were not regarded as feeling in the same way as their oppressors ; but as soon as the *emotional* realization of the position was forced on people, the system was condemned. It is probable that such a book as *Uncle Tom's*

[1] Pope is a classical literary instance of one who possessed such power. Because of it, he was our most venomous satirist.

Cabin had more effect in freeing the American slaves than hundreds of abstract arguments about justice and humanity ; and to-day it generally only needs a visit to a prison to convert quite self-satisfied citizens into ardent members of the Prison Reform League. The men and women in prison are so like ourselves, that we do not say, " there, but for the grace of God ", but rather, " there, but for sheer luck, sit I ", and wonder how it would feel if the luck changed. Then each item of prison life, dreary walls and rough clothes, hard beds, monotonous employment and degraded company acquire a piercing personal significance, and we shudder at the cruelty and unreason of the system. In the same way the modern humane feeling towards animals is due to the sympathetic imagination which realizes their feelings as though they were human. Modern poetry about animals shows this.[1] From such imaginative experience reforms spring. Hence an unprogressive society is generally one where barriers of class or custom isolate the experience of each section of the community.

(2) A second type of imagination is that which is concerned with material things. We image the dress we are making, but H. G. Wells imagined all the strange conveniences—many of them now actualities—which were enjoyed in the world of *The Sleeper Awakes*. So, too, imagination preceded the invention of the gramophone or wireless telephony, or of any of the revolutionary devices of modern days.

(3) The third type of imagination, which has a personal rather than a social use, is the imagination that is used simply for pleasure. This may take many forms. The child imagines that chairs are ships, or that bears will catch him if he walks on the lines and not the squares of paving stone,[2] and such fancies make life more amusing to him. The older child day-dreams of what he will do when he is grown up, or of some glorious day when, in front of a yelling crowd, he shoots the goal which wins the cup. The routine typist in the Underground reads Zane Grey, the comfortable academic person Thomas Hardy's *Tess*, while the parted lover murmurs, " How like a winter hath my

[1] Stephens, *The Snare* ; Hodgson, *The Bull*, etc.
[2] A. A. Milne, *When We Were Very Young*.

absence been." In all cases whether the imagination be our own or another's, we turn to it with pleasure and find through it an added satisfaction in life.

This need for imagination springs from various sources. To happiness it adds depth and richness by uniting to our immediate experience that of other minds, and by revealing aspects of things which we had not previously noticed, and which, when noticed, are found to be strangely beautiful. In discontent or boredom it affords an escape into a world in which we are strong, clever or successful, in sorrow we learn that others have suffered before us, and at all times we gain variety and the possibility of new experiences.

If, then, imagination has so much value for society and the individual it is important to encourage it during the period of education. A certain power of imagination is a natural gift in most people. In many children it is undesirably strong, leading them to see goblins in the shadows of trees, and to confuse fact with fiction to such a degree that they seem incapable of telling the truth as others know it.

This exuberance of imagination is usually checked as the child grows older, and efforts are then made to cultivate a tamer kind that shall be useful in composition lessons and not betray the owner into gross mis-statements of fact. It is necessary to help children to distinguish between fact and imagination, but it is not sensible to attempt to crush one manifestation of imagination and then cultivate another. The essential process is the same. What is needed is an imagination which works in and through reality. The imaginings of a small child take little account of probability; he is partly too ignorant, partly too careless to consider whether bears are likely to be hiding behind area railings, or whether you could build a house all of toffee and lollipops. The adult's imagination, on the other hand, is either concerned with possibility, or, if it moves into the realms of fairy story, provides itself with a new set of natural laws, which work nearly as rigidly as those we normally experience. When Alice nibbles her mushroom and grows taller, or shorter, the results, given that situation, are probable enough. Giants with seven-league boots which confer invisibility, though they outrage our generally accepted laws of the probable, yet, within the realm of " seven-league-bootedness ", behave quite reasonably.

This disciplining of the imagination by experience is even more important when the imagining concerns practical things. Nearly every mechanically minded child constructs in imagination, at some time or other, a machine for achieving perpetual motion ; the invention does not revolutionize the world because the inventor is too ignorant to make his invention a practical possibility. This type of imagination, if it is to bear fruit, must be combined with extensive knowledge.

Not only does experience refine and direct our natural imaginings, but it is in itself a *source* of imagination. It cannot confer imaginative powers on those who possess none by nature, but it can quicken what powers each possesses. A child brought up in one district without access to the outside world, and with poor facilities for broadening his experience through books, would have as a rule little power of imagination. He would not have the images in which to clothe his thoughts. He could not compare the model cottages of Bournville with the two-roomed hovels of his own colliery village, and imagine a district in which houses were an adornment and not a blot on the landscape ; nor could he go in imagination to the Indian Ocean and indulge in adventures which would supplement his " trivial round ".

We can all see for ourselves the effect which experience has on our imagination. The wildest fairy story we choose to invent is shot through and through with our own experience.

Beware then of expecting children of little experience of any kind to " imagine " scenes of which they have no knowledge. They need the elements with which they may build up their mental pictures. A teacher once found out that the only " cataract " slum children knew of was the eye disease of that name ! No wonder they could not imagine the scene described in " The splendour falls on castle walls . . . and the wild cataract leaps in glory." Good illustrations and vivid word pictures are the best way of enriching the child's mind and cultivating this imagination.

Though Wordsworth is wrong in his prose account of the

nature of imagination, he is right in the place he gives it among the qualifications of the poet, and the emphasis he lays on experience as one of its pre-conditions.   In the preface quoted above, he says that the qualities needed by a poet are : (1) observation, i.e., the ability to observe with accuracy things as they are in themselves.   (2) Sensibility—which the more exquisite it is, the wider will be the range of a poet's perceptions.   (3) Reflection which makes the poet acquainted with the value of actions . . . and assists the sensibility in perceiving their connection with each other. (4) Imagination and Fancy.   That is, a poet needs to be acutely sensitive to events around him.   He must notice the things of sight and sound and the emotions of himself and others ; then he must reflect on this experience until from such experience and reflection new imaginings are born. This is the relation of imagination to experience in the adult, who possesses imagination, and cares to refine and improve it by experience.

Imagination is not a power which we continually employ ; rather we use it by fits and starts as occasion demands. When we are setting off to walk down certain crowded streets to the draper's, there to buy a dozen dusters, we do not purposely give play to our imagination ; we are on business, and the jostle of the passing people keeps our attention fairly fixed.   But if by any chance we happen to hate walking through those streets and abominate the thought of buying dusters, which are to be used for spring cleaning, we may lapse into a day-dream and lose conscious perception of events round about us.   Again when teaching a class, we do not usually give our imagination much play—indeed, we may find it hard even to tell an imaginative story well ; but when we come home many of us sit down with a novel for half an hour after tea, or just indulge our own idle fancies.

On the whole, imagination provides for the individual either a means of escape or a relaxation.   The imagination in times of weariness is almost always of the unpractical kind.   It usually tends to give an imagined satisfaction of wishes which are denied fulfilment in ordinary life.   And because day-dreams allow us to gain some satisfaction, if only an unreal one, they hearten us for our other work.

The imaginings which aid us to escape from present reality, may be of all kinds. In minds of less experience and power they may be quite unpractical ; in others they may achieve coherent organization, and be closely connected with reality, but at a different point from that at which the imaginer actually is. One headmaster, who finds a school a none too pleasant responsibility, employs all his spare time in inventing improvements in wireless receiving sets. Many a clerk in a dreary office who spends his days writing " paid and unpaid ", may nourish many darling fancies which later are utilized in literary work. One remembers Charles Lamb in the India House ! Anthony Trollope, as a small boy, was despised by his schoolfellows and excluded from much of their school life. The result was that he must needs amuse himself. " As a boy, even as a child, I was thrown much upon myself. I have explained, when speaking of my schooldays, how it came to pass that other boys would not play with me. I was, therefore, much alone and had to form my plays within myself. Play of some kind was necessary to me then, as it has always been. Study was not my bent, and I could not please myself by being all idle. Thus it came to pass that I was always going about with some castle in the air firmly built within my mind. Nor were these efforts in architecture spasmodic, or subject to constant change from day to day. For weeks, months, if I remember rightly, from year to year, I would carry on the same tale, binding myself down to certain proportions and proprieties and unities. Nothing impossible was ever introduced—nor even anything which, from outward circumstances, would seem to be violently improbable. I myself was, of course, my own hero, such is the necessity of castle building, but I never became a king or a duke— much less when my height and personal appearance were fixed could I be an Antinous or 6ft. high. But I was a very clever person, and beautiful young women were fond of me." [1]

These " castles in the air " were a means of escape from the dullness and degradation of loafing about solitary among a crowd of playing companions ; they were also the satisfaction of desires natural to the growing boy—the love

[1] *Autobiography.*

of praise and the admiration of women ; they were kept in a certain conformity to reality and the canons of art by the developing richness of Trollope's genius. This day-dreaming was the foundation of his novel writing, yet he himself declares, " There can, I imagine, hardly be a more dangerous mental practice," and many " practical " people would say the same.

Day-dreaming is not in itself bad : on the contrary, it is, for many people, almost a condition of mental health ; it becomes dangerous under certain circumstances, or when carried to excess. In the first place day-dreaming often occupies much time which could be more profitably spent. It is physically better for a child to play games than to sit hunched up in a corner telling himself stories ; it is mentally better for a child to read an exciting story book than to pursue its own unformed imaginings. Sometimes the wishes which the day-dream satisfies are wholesome. An only child who gets too little of the companionship of children of her own age, frequently invents an imaginary play-mate, who shares her games and very often her meals or bed. The boy who loves authority, but is perhaps not actually able to exercise it, may spend many happy hours arranging the laws and customs of an imaginary kingdom ; but, in many cases, day-dreams take a less healthy turn, and the child broods over problems of sex or love, at an age when he possesses insufficient knowledge for a sane study of the subjects.

But thirdly, even when the topic of the day-dream is not unhealthy, since it involves a turning away from life, *excessive* indulgence in it may result in an impoverishment of experience and consequently may weaken active purpose, and cause the personality to become less wide and forceful. The youth who attempts to substitute imagination for real experience loses much ; and the man who is content to be successful in day-dreams, and does not care what happens in real life, is exposing himself to disaster.

An uncontrolled vivid imagination sometimes makes people cowards in practical affairs. An unpleasant situation, which they have to face in the future, becomes so real to them, and all its perils so clearly emphasized, that they quail before it ; whereas an unimaginative person comes freshly to the conflict, untried by the vivid " presentations " of it.[1]

It is, therefore, the *excess* and not the *fact* of day-dreaming which is dangerous, and the way to avoid these dangers is not to discourage imagination, but to bring it into contact with reality.

The imagination which abandons reality is often the flower of unhappiness. *Punch* has a story of a king who wished to have the perfect poet at his court. His messengers were sent out and discovered the poet starving in a garret and writing immortal verse. He was brought to the king, given a pension, servants and every comfort. His inspiration at once failed him, and it was not till he was cast into a dungeon, for failing to fulfil expectation, that he was once more able to write well. The king, being wise this time, kept him in misery all his days, and enjoyed the fame of being celebrated by the greatest poet of the world. The truth in this story is that poetry and the more emotional arts are the result of conflict and stress in the personality ; they do not reach their highest expression in the happy. Shelley had perhaps the ideal upbringing for the perfect imaginative poet, and the comparative dearth of great imaginative literature, in our day, may be in part due to the greater happiness of the bulk of the population. If one studies the writers who are more definitely imaginative in the narrower sense, such as Algernon Blackwood, the fact that imagination springs out of suffering is only too clear.[2]

From the educational point of view then, if we wish to discourage excessive day-dreaming and encourage children to employ their imagination in the service of reality, we must do so by making them happy in, and through reality. On the other hand, society esteems Shelley's verse as one of the most valuable possessions in the history of the world, and a novelist can make a very handsome living out of the demand for imaginative literature !

The fact is that all of us, at one time or another, wish to escape into strange worlds, and very few of us have the power to do it alone.

[1] V. R. H. Benson, *The Coward.*
[2] How do you account for the pessimistic imaginings of A. E. Housman ?

> Could I take me to some cavern for mine hiding,
> In the hill-tops where the sun scarce hath trod;
> Or a cloud make the home of mine abiding,
> As a bird among the bird-droves of God ! [1]

says the harassed chorus in the *Hippolytus*, and that wish is echoed every day by a large portion of the population. The poets and the novelists give them the magic carpets, open the gates of Damascus and let the caravan set out " along the golden road to Samarcand ". We demand from others what we cannot do for ourselves, for the world of Romance is like De la Mare's Arabia a " far " land and one

> Where the princes ride at noon,
> 'Mid the verdurous vales and thickets,
> Under the ghost of the moon ;
> And so dark is that vaulted purple
> Flowers of the forest rise
> And toss into blossom 'gainst the phantom stars
> Pale in the noonday skies.

It needs a very robust enjoyer of modern civilization, such as Kipling, to assure us that

> Romance brought up the nine-fifteen,

or a man very much at ease in the country to say

> The jonquils bloom round Samarcand—
> Maybe ; but lulled by Avon stream,
> By hawthorn-scented breezes fanned,
> 'Twere mere perversity to dream
> Of Samarcand. [2]

The most remarkable thing about the day-dream or the imagination of escape is the amount of money that people are prepared to spend on its enjoyment. The cinemas above all provide it to-day and in 1934 the British public spent £40,950,000 at the cinema. Next comes the magazine, the cheap novelette, the more serious novel, the theatre, poetry—this list is in ascending order of difficulty and decreasing popularity. It is easy to follow the story and enjoy the emotions of the cinema. Poetry is difficult and the emotions and day-dreams represented are less common

---

[1] Euripides, *Hippolytus*. Tr. by Murray.
[2] A. H. Bullen.

to mankind. But beautiful women, luxurious clothes and food, wild west adventures, unnaturally talented children all make a direct appeal to most people and allow them to identify themselves with someone on the screen and thus satisfy their desire for romance or adventure—the daydream is made more complete and entrancing by the details of the film star's lives that are published so lavishly. It suggests that most people find modesty, honesty and economy very irksome virtues when they hear so delightedly of the lack of them in others.

For children the importance of imagination is different. It takes a large part in the play of all normal children and develops as their minds develop. The small child, aged 2 or 3, plays a large number of games in which he is a " puffer-train ", an aeroplane, a lion or a ticket-collector. He is sometimes the milkman or the baker. When he is a little older he plays " houses and families ", " schools " or more occasionally " ships ". In all these games he seems to be experimenting with experience. Usually the things or persons represented are those which appear to the child as powerful or desirable. There is no doubt that the child broods much on large powerful machines, and this interest remains with the boy till well in his 'teens as his drawing shows. He is also much impressed in his youth by the rôle of conductor or ticket-collector, and he probably thinks that the milkman or baker are powerful agents in distribution.

In " homes and families " or " school " he is again experimenting with experience, and again usually, if he can, takes the important position, leaving his younger brothers and sisters, or the family dolls to fill the inferior rôles. Frequently he arms himself with all the traditional, and often unexperienced might of his position, and the child who has been most kindly treated in school plays the brutal pedagogue with a cane.

This play undoubtedly helps the child to endure some of the difficulties of childhood, and when the difficulties are more acute the play may become more specific. A child's wishes may become clear in his " imaginative " drawing. If he hates his father, he pictures him chained and in gaol. If he is frightened of horses he draws himself riding one and thus tries to establish an imaginative mastery over the dreadful beast. The child is not able, frequently, to think in words, and these images serve as the vehicles of his thought, and their externalization helps him to get control of the situation and himself.

A special development of this early imagination continues with some children in their constructive games. Some children at the age of 8 or 9 take to the unimaginative intricacies of Meccano, but others absolutely refuse the game and prefer plasticine or building blocks. The purpose of this choice is to obtain a material with which they can express their thoughts. On their little stage they play out an elaborate commentary on various aspects of life as they know it. They build harbours and docks and discuss, as they go, all the functions of locks, cranes or sheds. One child pursued, day after day, the fortunes of a village which had a complicated economic life, a variety of inhabitants, an army, a war and a post-war housing problem. Into the game he put his speculation on banking, national finance, army training, the reasons for war, and the problem of disorder. The boy was 10, and some of the solutions of the problems were very ingenious. The fascination that the game had for him was obvious, and he returned from his imagined world as unwillingly as the adolescent from his novel.

This aspect of imagination is one of the reasons for the extreme importance of the free use of constructive materials by children which has been referred to before.

FOR DISCUSSION

1.—Madame Montessori asserts that fairy stories are bad for children. Argue for and against this statement.
2.—Describe methods you have seen used to train the imagination. Of what value do you think these are ?
3.—Describe how you would give children the materials with which to imagine the scene in :
    The Listeners, by De La Mare.
    As You Like It, by Shakespeare.
    The Forsaken Merman, by Arnold.
    Kubla Khan, by Coleridge.
4.—Imagine a fairy story. Then analyse its scenes and events and trace their origin in your mind, thus showing how you use your experiences for new inventions ; or choose an author of whose life you know something, and attempt to show how much of his

work is experience and how much imagination (e.g., compare Wordsworth's poems with Dorothy Wordsworth's journal).

5.—For your own satisfaction write out one of your day-dreams, and see how far it is a fulfilment of your desires.

6.—What would you do in oral composition lessons to develop and direct the imaginative powers of children of 10 years ?

7.—How would you set about helping an " only " child of 8 years who found school life difficult and who took refuge in persistent day-dreaming ?

BOOKS

GEORGE H. GREEN, *The Day Dream.*

*ALGERNON BLACKWOOD, *Episodes before Thirty.*

*ANTHONY TROLLOPE, *Autobiography.*

*EMILE LAUVRIÈRE, *La Vie d'Edgar A. Poe.*

*These three books show different types of imagination at work.

DICKENS, *Pickwick* and *David Copperfield.* These are the two most autobiographical of Dickens' novels. They are also perhaps the best.

GALTON, *Inquiries Into Human Faculty.* Essay on Mental Imagery. This essay records the first investigation into the subject.

R. GRIFFITHS, *Imagination in Early Childhood.*

CHAPTER XVI

WORDS AND THOUGHT—I

" What's in a name ? "

In an earlier chapter, on perception, we discussed the manner in which we come to perceive " objects " and the way in which, when we have perceived the object, we give it a name which symbolizes the whole complex of qualities we associate with it. Thus it comes to pass that words are frequently used to take the place of images in our mental processes, and in some people are almost invariably employed to the exclusion of visual, or other imagery, of the thing itself. Before, however, this can happen freely, we have to make certain generalizations. Every common noun we use is the name, not of one particular thing, but of a class of things, and is so used in thought ; but these things are sufficiently similar, for our purposes, to be treated as a unity ; when they are not, we sub-divide the class or give proper names. To take an example : we refer to the general class " dog " when we say, " I hate dogs " ; but on other occasions it is necessary to divide in greater detail, as when we say, " I want to have a terrier." A dog fancier has to be yet more precise and distinguish different breeds of terriers, while on occasions he must know enough of particular dogs to estimate the value of a pedigree. If then, in what follows, we say that a general or universal term is employed, and that we generalize a class of objects, it must be understood that the size and inclusiveness of the class generalized depend on particular circumstances. This, however, makes no difference to the principle involved.

This process of generalization, or the formation of the concept of a class of objects has often been treated as a mystery by the metaphysicians. They have imagined that because we use a common noun " chair ", which includes many particular and individual chairs and yet *is* not any one of them, that there must be some entity corresponding to the common noun. Plato's Theory of Ideas was the first and most famous solution of this problem. This theory was that there was some entity which corresponded to the common noun, and that individual things acquired their particular characteristics through " participation " in the nature of this entity. These entities were not included in the material world, but existed on some " ideal " plane which could be apprehended by thought but not by sense. Thus there was an " ideal " table which gave to all material tables that quality of being-a-table which entitled them to be included under a common name ; and there was an " ideal " beauty which was partially reflected in all the different objects of beauty in the world of sense.

Psychologically, this metaphysical problem has little excuse. As far as we are concerned, the important thing is to discover how we come to form these class concepts, not whether, when formed, they refer to any one individual thing. The process is easier to describe than to explain, and is one which occurs at all periods of life, though doubt- less, like all our most important intellectual achievements, it occurs most extensively in childhood. We will take an example from adult life because, since our introspective powers are greater when we are grown up, we are more consciously aware of how we tackle mental problems. Suppose we have a botanical friend. On several occasions she tells us that certain flowers, differing considerably in size or growth, are Veronicas. We may, in spite of this, remain ignorant of the exact botanical structure of this order and be unable to say whether the flower is epigynous or hypogynous or whether it has two or more aborted stamens. All the same, when, a little later, a flower is shown us and we are asked to name its species, we may at once say " Veronica " ; and if asked our reasons, say " It looked like it." This means that from our knowledge of particular flowers we have formed a generalized conception of the characteristics of the order, and this conception, though not exact in a scientific sense, is sufficient to allow us to refer new specimens to the class. It is interesting to notice how rapidly such generalizations can be formed. We can recognize a natural order in botany with outstanding characteristics after seeing only one or two specimens ; other orders may be much harder to recognize. In our practised recognition we forget how inarticulate our methods of recognition are. If we look at a tree in a winter hedgerow and say " that is an elm ", how few of us could give in words, or even draw *accurately* on paper the characteristics by which we recognize it. We have a wordless vague scheme of " elm tree " in our mind and the visual experience of this tree fits it.

The definitions of the old grammar or spelling book are, therefore, unpsychological in that they try to make definite things which can quite conveniently be left vague, and to burden the mind with useless knowledge, often inexact. The true definition of most manufactured things is in terms of use, and small children invariably give definitions of this kind. A spoon is " something to eat soup with ", a pencil " something to draw with "; it is useless to complicate this definition by inserting such descriptions as " an implement made of wood " or metal, or sometimes bone or ivory.

The case is different in the realm of abstract ideas, which are often very confused and yet influence conduct in a most pronounced way. The discovery of the exact meaning of abstract ideas, such as justice, temperance and courage, was one of the aims that Socrates set himself. The most famous of the Platonic dialogues, *The Republic*, grows up round the question, " What is Justice ? " Plato considers the definitions " Giving every man his due ", and " The interest of the stronger ", explains and refutes them, making the final suggestion that justice is the " correct performance of function ", both in the state and in the soul of the individual. It is important for morals to have such definitions, if conduct is to be guided by anything but blind adherence to custom ; and it is good for individuals to know what they mean when they condemn the practices of their neighbours as " superstitious " or " barbarous ".

The process by which words obtain their full meaning is gradual, and for most of us a large number of the words in use have only vague meanings attached to them ; but so long as we are content to use our words strictly within the province in which we have learnt them, we can be fairly safe. Take some of the flowers of which poets speak—galingale, amaranth and asphodel. We could not write a botanical description of these. All we can assert is that galingale grows in meadows near streams ; that amaranth and moly grow near together, and are good to lie on [1] ; that asphodel grows in the Islands of the Blest, and is presumably one of the most beautiful Greek flowers. There is a bird, the bittern, which haunts the marshes of poesy ; and strange boats, caravels and junks, sail the seas of romance ; while Tibetans shoot with " jingals from a jong " at invading troops. We discover the meaning of these and other words by a process of the same sort by which we learn to give one name to a number of different objects. We perform an unwitting comparison of examples, and the larger the number of examples we meet, the more accurate will be our knowledge of the word—even if we cannot give a definition in dictionary style. From a single example we can conclude little. A psychologist records that, during the early days of the war, he heard the statement " this balloon has too many gadgets ", and when asked a few days later what a " gadget " was, he promptly replied " part of a balloon ". The following is an extract from an article which appeared in the *Westminster Gazette* during 1924, and is typical of many paragraphs which appeared about that time. Try to conclude what a " putsch " is from the extract, and then look the word up in a German dictionary.

" There was much conflicting news yesterday about the Rhineland ' Putsch '. While Treves, Bonn and Wiesbaden were added to the list of separatist towns, it appears that the Rhenish party have been driven from control in Aix-la-Chapelle."

The educational conclusion to be drawn from all this is that the royal road to a large and exact vocabulary lies through abundance of reading, not through lists of words on the blackboard, and exercises inviting the pupil to " put the following words into sentences ". These lessons are better

[1] V. *The Lotus Eaters*, Tennyson.

than nothing, but they are far less efficient for the enriching of vocabulary than interesting silent reading for the same amount of time.

The convenience of words for thought is so great that it has often been doubted whether we could think at all if we had no words. Introspection will tell us that it is quite possible to think without words. As we lie in bed at night visual images of scenes pass before our eyes, and we very often come to conclusions concerning them. This process might well be described as the work of thought, yet it does not involve the use of words. If we believe that animals think—and to judge by appearances some animals such as cats and dogs and monkeys do think—they must think without the use of words.

However this may be, words are a very great assistance to thought :

(i) By indicating all the qualities of an object, not only those which are obvious to one sense, e.g., sight, they render easier the consideration of that object from different aspects.

(ii) By means of words we think of concepts which correspond with objects not present to the senses, e.g., we can think of infinity, eternity, virtue, charity as abstract entities, irrespective of particular instances of virtue or charity. When the words have led to the formation of these general concepts an image may be aroused in our minds when we think of the word or the concept, but it is unlikely that most of us would form the concept at all if it were not for the existence of a word.

(iii) The third great use of words is that they make permanent and communicable the results of thought. If we had no words we could not communicate many of our thoughts to others, nor could we describe any remote object, nor, if our thoughts concerned any but practical things, could we perpetuate them. In the days before language, a craftsman could devise a new method of making a club, and teach the other members of the tribe to do it in the same way, but he could not pass on to others his speculations about the stars or the sun. It is only necessary to spend a few days in a country of which we do not know the language to realize how completely dependent we are on words for the communication of all but the simplest thoughts. So long as we can convey our meaning by pointing all goes well, but if we want to ask whether it will be fine to-morrow, we are helpless.

Thus, although we can think without words, words are a great assistance for all thought, and are indispensable for certain kinds of thought ; so that very roughly the range of our thoughts varies with the size of our vocabulary. New words may introduce us to new ideas or give meaning and precision to old ones ; but they will only do this when connected with the sense impressions to which they ultimately refer. There is, then, a certain amount of justification both for those who devote attention to the teaching of words (as did the old teachers who were supposed to have been swept away by Pestalozzi's reforms, but whose teaching lasted on in another form in his object lessons), as well as for those who claim that all true learning must be based on direct contact with the real thing.

The fact is that there are at least two stages in the learning of words—that in which the little child learns to connect common words with the objects and qualities to which they refer, and that in which the older child is able by analogy to pass on to the meaning of new words which refer to things outside his experience. For example, direct experience is necessary for a small child to form a reasonably correct idea of snow, and children brought up in snowless countries are wildly excited when they experience their first snow storm. But, given a knowledge of snow and a photograph, it is possible to form a faint—though only a faint—idea of a Swiss winter.

In thought, therefore, we largely employ words, but can also think in images, and the nature of the thought is not seriously affected by the instruments through which it is carried out. We can consider, then, the act of thought without further reference to the means employed in it.

In its origin, thought may be described as a supplement to instinct, and it is employed when any difficulty or change in the circumstances renders the normal functioning of an instinct difficult or impossible. When we act instinctively there is " no time to think ", and action follows immediately on the impulse that gives rise to it. In a similar way habitual action proceeds without thought, and very often would be hindered if made the object of thought. You would probably fall off your bicycle if you thought out each movement required in riding it. All our habitual bad habits such as biting our nails proceed unwittingly. Many useful habits may be performed at the wrong time through want of thought. For example, many people, when they change their clothes in the middle of the day, find themselves winding up their watches as if they were going to bed.

Thought arises when there is some obstacle to our normal habitual or instinctive action. If we experience some change in circumstances which renders a modification of behaviour necessary, we notice this necessity for thought very clearly. Suppose that we alter our method of doing our hair, what was before a perfectly habitual process, accomplished while we thought of some entirely different subject, becomes now a matter which requires thought on each occasion. So too with instinctive actions. Our instincts would perhaps lead us to attack a person who makes us angry ; but circumstances prevent this attack. We, therefore, " think out " how we can deal with the situation in some manner which does not infringe our social code.

It has been argued [1] that thought is itself an instinct. It is certainly natural for most of us to think, and we require no teaching to perform the simpler mental processes. If we define an instinct merely as an innate tendency to a certain mode of behaviour, thought is instinctive. If, however, Professor McDougall's definition of instincts is accepted, then thought cannot be called instinctive since it has no *specific* stimulus nor emotion. The question, however, is mainly one of terminology.

The condition which gives rise to thought is, roughly, the consciousness of a problem. For example, if some action is checked, which we yet desire to perform, we are faced with the problem of our future behaviour and think out the means of attaining our end. Thus, by enabling us to vary our actions, thought prevents that comparative fixity of instinctive behaviour which was mentioned earlier. The power to think is, therefore, one of the great signs of intelligence.

[1] Graham Wallas, *The Great Society.*

In a primitive act of thought there are three parts : 1, the apprehension of a situation ; 2, tentative suggestions for meeting the difficulty ; and 3, action in accordance with some course that has been thought of. We may give these stages other names and call them apprehension, hypothesis and verification. The last two terms are used when scientific method is being discussed.

The first part of the process, that of apprehension, appears easy at first sight ; but when we really bring our minds to bear on them, most problems present quite unexpected difficulties. The problem of planting a flower bed with seedlings may at first appear simple, but when we come to consider the matter closely, apprehension of the *complete* situation is by no means easy. The colours of the different flowers must harmonize, and we must, therefore, know them. What are the dates of flowering of the various plants ? Which grow tall and which short ? Which thrive best near a wall and which away from it ? Soon we find that it is by no means easy to apprehend all the factors involved in the problem. Expert knowledge—though it may help the solution—often increases the apparent difficulty of a task. It is for this reason that angels walk more warily than fools. Many people, who amuse themselves by inventing problems they would like to have to solve, find unexpected difficulties in the details. Some plan the perfect house, a few get so far as to try to put their plans on paper. At once a host of difficulties springs up—stairs will not fit in, doors and chimneys get in each other's way, corridors lack windows. Only an architect probably could apprehend *all* the conditions of the problem and so devise a successful solution !

The second part of the process, the suggestion of a tentative solution, or hypothesis, is one of the most interesting and perhaps one of the most obscure in this branch of psychology. Where do our ideas come from ? Some are undoubtedly due to memory and are suggested by analogy from some partially similar situation which we remember. Some are suggested directly by objects round us, as when we stand in front of a shop wondering what we should buy for supper, and a tin of salmon catches our eye. But others ? What made Francis Thompson think of the metaphor contained in the title of the *Hound of Heaven* ? What suggested to Dumas the characters of his four famous friends—Athos, Porthos, Aramis and D'Artagnan ? What put into Epstein's mind his conception of Christ ? What exactly made Newton suggest the theory of gravitation as the solution of certain phenomena which puzzled him ? It is almost impossible to say. None of these ideas were absolutely new in the sense of having *no* analogy with anything in the world, but they were *comparatively* new ; they are true works of imagination, and in only one mind out of millions would experience of life bear such fruit.

The source from which these ideas spring seems to be little under volitional control. We cannot force ourselves to have ideas, and much deliberate thinking tends to check rather than increase the supply. For this reason, worry (the continual recurrence to the mind of a problem it cannot solve, accompanied by a feeling of fear) is the most unlikely state in which to escape one's difficulties. Sleep is a wonderful aid in solving problems. Occasionally a solution actually occurs in the form of a dream and many children have, at one time or another, dreamt the answer to a problem in geometry or algebra ; but more often when we wake up and return to a consideration of the problem, the solution suggests itself at once. This is partly due to the absence of fatigue, but also partly, it seems, to some process that went on in sleep. The most famous instance of this is described in Stevenson's " Chapter on Dreams ",[1] in which he tells how, when his bank balance was low, he could generally dream the plot of a story. These plots were often suitable, and one at least has become famous— that of *Dr. Jekyll and Mr. Hyde.*

If sleep is not convenient, the best method of solving a problem is to allow the mind to remain comparatively blank and to wait for something to turn up. This process can be aided by various devices. The following is a trick for inventing plots for plays or stories, which, if it does not produce masterpieces, has rarely failed to produce something. You decide roughly on the type of thing required, e.g., a play on Bonnie Prince Charlie. Then you make yourself comfortable in an easy chair or on a bed, banish all

[1] In the volume *Across the Plains.*

worries of the day from your mind, and write down one after the other a list of disconnected words just as they occur to you—ship, light, town, soldier, girl, marriage—or what not. When you have about a dozen words you stop, consider them for a while, and suddenly a plot—a combination of the words and events—occurs to you. It may need much manipulating before it will fit the stage, but it is there—something at least to work on—a beginning !

This faculty of invention differs very markedly in different people. Some are always ready to suggest a course of action in any difficulty, others stand agape and cannot proceed at the smallest mishap. It is interesting to notice how long we sometimes are in devising the simplest solutions. We may gaze for a long time at a bar of Meccano which is too long for the place into which we wish to fit it, before it occurs to us to allow an end to stick out somewhere. We may debate the possibility of making jam in all the utensils in the house, before we remember that our neighbour has a pan that would suit our purpose excellently, and that she is willing to lend. Chess is a game in which this process of thought, with its successes and failures, can be studied almost indefinitely.

Lastly, we have the process of verification, either in action or in images. In a simple and unimportant matter we may at once carry out our idea in action, and find out if it is right or wrong by our success or failure ; but in more important matters we usually take more care. We may try out our suggested scheme of action in images and attempt to see from them what will happen in practice. We may make plans or drawings, models, or all kinds of preliminary experiments.

In science this verification is a most important step. Certain phenomena may occur, a hypothesis may be invented to cover them ; but that by no means ends the process ; the hypothesis must be verified, it must be shown to explain the facts in a way which no other one so far thought of does, and it must be capable, if circumstances allow, of being used for the prediction of similar phenomena. It is said of Newton that when he had thought of his formula for gravitation he worked out from it various positions of the moon. On comparing his positions with the records of observations he found discrepancies. He therefore concluded that his formula was wrong, and laid it aside for ten years. At the end of that period a new set of observations was published correcting the former. These did agree with the calculations, and Newton now considered his formula proved. This attitude of suspended judgment and delayed action is not easy, and much of a scientist's training is devoted—indirectly—to producing the frame of mind which will submit its hypothesis to careful verification. The average man does not do this. If an explanation appears to cover the facts it is taken as true, even if it is only one of many which at first sight would do so equally well.

In education we are concerned to some extent in teaching children to verify results and to compare opinions with facts. This can be done in every lesson where the children are asked to suggest solutions for problems of various kinds, but especially is the process taught in lessons such as nature study, in which children can be asked to form opinions, e.g., as to the growth of seeds, and then to check their opinions by their observations. The same attitude of mind can be cultivated to a certain extent, though less easily, in the more literary subjects ; and the older children could be taught a little of the rudiments of historical criticism and encouraged in a small way to compare authorities. Much, however, is gained if the importance of this attitude of mind is merely suggested to them.

On the general question of arousing thought in schools, we come back to the position of an earlier chapter. Thought, like other mental processes, is purposive. It must be aroused by some problem, and, if possible, one connected with a real purpose. If we cannot satisfy these requirements, we must still invent problems for the children to solve and endow them with such derivative interest as we can manage. It is one of the merits of the Dalton Plan that its well-planned assignments readily present themselves to the children as problems to be solved, rather than as so many facts to be memorized.

WORDS AND THOUGHT

FOR DISCUSSION

1.—Give a description of a dog, cat and horse such that one who had never seen any of these animals might know to which order a given animal belonged.
2.—Read a dialogue of Plato e.g., *Meno*, or *Phædrus*, and then construct a Socratic dialogue to elicit a definition of " Superstition ".
3.—Without using a dictionary give a definition of " precinct ", " drink " (verb), " etching ", " jazz ".
4.—Play the following game—Sir Walter Raleigh's Word and Question game in *From a Cloud*—and analyse the thought processes involved. Let three or more people play. Each writes a word on one slip of paper and a question on another, e.g., *Word*, Death ; *Question*, " Who rang the bell ? " Then the slips are shuffled and each player takes one word and one question. Each must write a set of verses answering the question and containing the word.
5.—Do you consider a doubting mind a valuable asset ? Consider different conditions and types of doubt.

BOOKS

JOHN DEWEY, *How We Think*. A useful discussion of the whole question of thought.
MARRIOTT, *Exercises in Thinking and Expression*. A text book for use with older children. The exercises are directed to improving the use of words and the simpler processes of reasoning.
JACK LONDON, *Before Adam*. This novel brings out clearly the disadvantages of having no language.

CHAPTER XVII

THOUGHT—II

" Then join you with them, like a rib of steel,
To make strength stronger."

THE primitive type of thought described in the last chapter is adequate for a simple type of life where action is motivated directly by needs, but it is rapidly left behind when needs of a more complicated kind arise. As civilization progresses a double change takes place. The individual learns to employ a less fitful mode of thinking and one which is less dependent on immediate needs and problems ; and secondly, groups of men learn to unite for purposes of thought, not only for action.

The educated adult generally has two distinct methods of thought at his disposal. There is the method already described which is adapted to dealing with a problem, and which is by its nature uncertain and unsuitable when rigid time limits are imposed ; and there is the other method, which consists in steady mental application to a task, comparatively simple, but which can only be accomplished by prolonged mental effort. As examples we can take the act of thought by which we solve a difficult geometrical problem, and the steady plodding which takes us through several pages of moderately easy Latin translation. Eminent mathematicians, such as Poincaré, have recorded that some of their best solutions have occurred to them when right away from their work : and, as we all learnt at school, the easiest way to deal with a hard problem is to leave it alone for a while and hope that the solution will occur to us ; no school boy, on the other hand, ever managed his construe in this manner. He may reserve a particularly difficult passage for later consideration—and he would be wise to do so—but the bulk of the task must be done by steady effort. This latter type of thinking is what mainly distinguishes the educated man from one who has received a poor scholastic training. There are many men who can scythe grass or carry stones for an eight hours' day, without being unduly fatigued, yet if they are asked to do an hour or two of mental work of similar difficulty, e.g., adding up figures or drafting letters, they are as helpless before it as the clerk would be at the prospect of a day's coal-getting.

A large part of the school course has, as an ultimate aim, to teach the child this controlled continuous type of thought, since, unless he learns it, he is unfitted for any but manual occupations. We do not understand the genesis of this type of thought sufficiently well to teach it directly, but we exact tasks from the child which call for its exercise, and in most cases the child learns for himself to think in the required way. A danger, however, sometimes arises when men and women, who have been forced into this way of thought without realizing its nature or its limitations, come to regard it as the only form of thought, and to label those who think in another way as lazy. This attitude is bad for everybody. Not all problems can be solved in an office chair, and the attempt to solve them in this way wastes time and energy. Very often the most truly industrious thing to do is to lay aside one's work and take a walk or a hot bath, and then resume, fresher and more inventive. Further, when these worshippers of " industry " and " application " are put in places of command, they cannot tolerate in others habits of work which differ from their own, and they are apt to make unjustifiable charges against the industry of their more intelligent subordinates ; thus causing much unhappiness and even ill health.

For efficient thinking both types of thought are required, though the proportions in which they are required vary in different callings. A poet is probably at one end of the scale. His works are the result of spontaneous invention rather than of persistent industry. Then, perhaps, comes the playwright, then the painter, then the novelist. The last has so much sheer manual work in writing the thirty to a hundred thousand words necessary for a novel, that at times he must almost feel himself a clerk. All these workers, because they are to some extent dependent on fitful invention, the " industrious " man is apt to regard as " lazy ". At the other end of the scale are administrators, teachers, librarians, business men, and all types of clerks and routine workers. The simpler the work, and the more monotonous it is, the less invention is required, and the greater is the element of mere assiduity. It is worth noting that the believer in the universal efficacy of " industry " is nearly always an " iron-bound " teacher or a business man. The clerks are not articulate, and the superior administrator is too clever to make so elementary a psychological mistake.

The second development of thought is that of co-operative thought, and this is rendered necessary by the complicated character of the problems which civilized man has to solve. The business man or the statesman must deal with problems in very distant countries—such as the conditions of growing rubber on the Congo, or the state of feeling in the Punjab. In many cases a solution, to be successful, must involve an amount of technical knowledge such as no individual is likely to possess. For example, in putting up a big new building the services of architect, contractor, electrician, heating expert, and many others, are needed [1] ; or in planning a campaign, the special needs and problems of the infantry, air force, transport, artillery, sappers, R.A.M.C., and the rest all have to be considered. In consequence of this the conditions of a successful solution are so complicated that any one man is very unlikely to remember them all. He may remember, to revert to our example of the house, the drains, and forget the damp course. Naturally, practice and expert knowledge will render it easier to keep all these conditions in mind, but even some good architects will put the larder on the south of the house in a place where it is bound to get too much heat.

These different complications of thought are dealt with in different ways. The difficulty raised by the remoteness of the problem is met by the organization of a regular supply of information. The ordinary man must trust largely to the newspapers for the data on which to argue about politics,

[1] The L.C.C., when erecting a recent building, seem to have neglected to take the advice of an expert in acoustics !

or the state of trade, or the condition of Russia. The correctness of his conclusions depend almost entirely on the reliability of the information received, and it is common knowledge that each newspaper deliberately distorts even such truth as it knows, to suit the interests behind it, or to flatter what it believes to be the prejudices of the class it serves.

More exalted or influential persons can pay for special investigators, and deputations may be sent out to make special reports, such as those furnished to the Labour Party on the subject of Russia. Even here there is no certainty that the facts are " correct ". Each man sees what he wishes to see, or is predisposed by previous thought to see. The different records of eye-witnesses in Russia, Germany and Austria just after the Great War illustrated this very clearly. Some reported famine, others abundance—and this though they had stayed in the same town at approximately the same time. The fact was, that the large hotels —catering for foreigners—and the principal streets were sufficiently well to do, but the faces of the ragged children in the parks told a different tale to anyone who looked for it.

When the problem is too complicated to be solved by an individual, some form of committee is frequently employed. The ultimate responsibility for some decision or other depends on one man, but he calls to his council the various experts concerned, and asks their opinion of the plan and the steps which their department will take to carry it out. In such cases it is necessary to evolve a rule of procedure so that each person may know what is expected of him. In some committees it is customary for each man to speak when he has something to say ; in others, the opinion of every man is asked in turn, either starting with the most influential, as in the Roman senate, or with the most junior, as in the Navy to-day. If all the members are not clear as to the mode of procedure to be adopted, much valuable information may be lost, through people waiting to be asked to speak when the chairman expected them to " butt in ".[1]

In other cases, a rigid demarcation of function is possible,

[1] Cf. the account of the sitting of the Dardanelles Committee in *Our Social Heritage,* by Graham Wallas.

and spheres of duty are allotted to the respective experts, who are then left to carry on their work in their own sphere more or less in their own way.

Another variation of this type of thought occurs in the systems of checking or revision employed by such bodies as the civil service, the Bank of England, or a fairly large college. Cases requiring decision are passed from hand to hand, and the decisions are revised by different people. In a college a simple case of this kind occurs when the education lecturer draws up a list of students for school practice, gives it to the secretary, who counts and checks it, and passes it on to the principal for further consideration and ultimate signature. In an institution such as the British Museum or the Bank of England, slips which one clerk has drawn up are revised by another to ensure correctness.

In this way defects of individual thought are remedied, fresh aspects of the matter are brought under consideration, and the conditions, some of which, if numerous, might escape one man's thought, are all or almost all taken into consideration.

Co-operative thought of this nature is by no means easy. It involves powers of judgment and organization, as well as a certain attitude of mind. In order to use profitably the information provided by others, it is necessary to have a certain power of judging the character of those who supply the information and also their probable prejudices. Before one can work well on a committee it is necessary to understand the common methods of procedure of such bodies. This knowledge is supposed to be so general that a society will ask anybody who can write to act as secretary, and anyone who is moderately influential to be chairman. The result is often chaos and indecisive meetings of interminable length. Those who have suffered from meetings of this nature will realize that chairmanship is an art which needs to be learnt, and which some persons are constitutionally incapable of acquiring. The rudiments of it can, and should be, taught in school. In that way much of the public time would be saved.

The problems connected with the revision of work depend more for their solution on mental attitude. The natural man tends to lose his temper when his work is criticized.

He tends to be tenaciously devoted to his own ideas and scornful of another's. In co-operation this must be changed —your own ideas must be as impartially treated as your colleague's, and his ideas receive as favourable consideration as your own. The situation may be complicated by all sorts of personal relations. When revision is a matter of formal office routine it is one thing ; when a superior, whom you suspect of jealousy, nips in the bud schemes on which your heart is set, it is almost impossible not to give way to resentment. Very intimate co-operation, as between husband and wife over the upbringing of children, or between two persons over the writing of a single book, is possible only if there is mutual confidence. Otherwise, quarrels are almost inevitable. A single piece of bad proof-reading may wreck any chance of future collaboration !

We must, therefore, when we find ourselves in a position where collaboration is necessary—as it is, for example, in all teaching posts—consider carefully how it may be best achieved, and what attitude of mind will most conduce to harmony and efficiency.

So far, in this and the last chapter, we have discussed thought that is essentially purposive. Not all thought, however, has this purposive quality to the same degree, for very often we are not conscious of any purpose in our thinking. The most conspicuous examples of this apparently purposeless thought are idle reverie and day-dreams. When we sit idly, or settle down to sleep, our minds are often occupied by flitting thoughts which seem to follow each other by mere association. Our thoughts slip from the misty view of chimneys outside our window to a picture of mist which a friend owned, to another picture which she herself painted, to the armistice celebration which that picture commemorated, to the war and so on. The length of such trains of thought would seem to vary in different people. In some minds they are short, obtruding themselves suddenly into periods of purposeful thought, or occupying the semi-idle periods when we are walking or bathing— other people seem to give themselves up to this type of thinking for longer periods.

If we take the trouble to record the contents of such thought periods we shall often find that the mind is mumbling over dry bones of memory rather than progressing to anything new. Very often the period has been occupied, or the train of thought initiated by scraps of poetry which we know by heart. Many people have a fairly large stock of such poems or songs, and these, in whole or part, are always floating in and out of their thoughts. On other occasions it is old conversations which pass through our minds, and we remake our successful jokes or re-utter our stinging repartees. When we grow too old to keep these things as mere thoughts, we become like the garrulous old bore who is for ever relating how he was " too good for Lord X " at that famous meeting at Y. It is humiliating to realize the poverty of our mental stock-in-trade, and one is sometimes tempted to believe with the Behaviourists that " thought is only the functioning of language mechanism ".[1]

There may be a purpose behind these flitting thoughts, but it is hard to discover—it is far easier to discover the purpose underlying day-dreams. In essence, as was said before, they afford an emotional satisfaction, and the aim is not a practical, but an emotional one. Whereas purposive thought is occupied largely with discovering means to an end, day-dreaming disregards the means and directs its attention to the end which it imagines as achieved.

In thought, processes of two kinds are involved which can be described in terms of logic as deduction and induction, if the emphasis is laid on the *exposition* of the thought ; or as the "education of correlates" or the "education of relations",[2] if the thought *process* is under consideration.

The process of deduction or the education of correlates consists essentially in apprehending a relationship and finding terms which fit that relation. As formulated in deduction it takes the form of the syllogism—

(*a*) All men are mortal.

S. is a man
∴. S. is mortal.

[1] Cf. J. B. Watson, *Psychology from the Standpoint of a Behaviourist.*
[2] Spearman, *Nature of Intelligence.*

As it appears in experimental psychology, the process consists in finding a fourth term to complete a proportion—

(b) As foot is to leg, so is hand to ?

or, Benevolent : malevolent :: deceitful : ?

The two examples are not exactly parallel, since in (b) we start one stage farther back than we did in (a). In the syllogism we start with the general principle, but in (b) we have to find that as well. From the two terms, foot and hand, we arrive at a general idea of their being parts of a limb, and then we bring the other part, hand and arm, under the same relation.

Induction, or the education of relations, is the first part of the process represented by the psychological test of analogies given above. From a number of instances a general rule or relation is discovered. In its logical form it can be symbolized.

x and y and z are white

x and y and z are all the swans on the lake

∴ all the swans on the lake are white.

In almost any real act of thought, we have, as in the analogies test, both types of process. We arrive at a principle and then proceed to apply it to the particular problem that we have in hand at the moment.

In most cases of everyday life the general principle is arrived at on evidence which would not satisfy the logician. To be formally valid an induction must contain a *complete* enumeration of all the possible cases—if it does not, an exception may be discovered later—as in the famous example of the swans. " All swans are white " was a generalization universally accepted until Australia was discovered ; then the time-honoured principle became untrue. In actual thought we form our generalizations on one or quite a few instances. This is especially so with children whose general knowledge and power of judgment are small.

A small boy who had hitherto worn his hair in curls was one day told that now he was growing up he must have it cut short. He burst into tears and begged to be allowed to keep his locks. His mother allowed a week to elapse and returned to the subject, to be met again by tears. On the third attempt she pressed him for the reason of his objection.

" Oh, Mummy," he sobbed, " if you cut my hair, I shall lose all my strength—*like Samson.*" He had generalized from one instance. Such stories of children abound : we laugh at them and forget that we commit the same fallacy every time we argue : " I knew a girl who got her feet wet and did not change her stockings, and so fell ill with pneumonia and died. Now you change your wet stockings or you will get pneumonia and die," or more briefly : " Jones was a rascal and a Socialist, therefore, all Socialists are rascals." On the other hand we may be quite right : " Tibby, our cat, likes milk ∴ all cats like milk ∴ I will offer this little stray cat milk." But an exactly similar form of reasoning may be false owing to our ignorance of some relevant fact which only special knowledge could reveal ; e.g., " Tom when he is hungry wants a large meal. This man, who has been starved for days, is *very* hungry ∴ he wants a very large meal." Such a large meal might kill the recipient.

The distinction of deduction and induction, and the formal arrangement of the syllogism, do not, therefore, correspond closely with our actual thought. They are, as they were originally intended to be, rather modes of exposition of a thought already formed. No form of exposition is really clearer than the syllogism, nor is there any which allows fallacies to be more easily detected. Very many plausible arguments at once disclose their falsity when thrown into syllogistic form ; for example, that famous argument, " I never did that when I was a boy," can be shown to depend on the implied premise, " I am perfection," which is a statement few men would have the audacity to make openly. It is a good plan, therefore, to arrange our ideas for exposition in the syllogistic form, though it is not usual to think in it.

It is also a good method of checking the most common of all fallacies, that called in formal logic affirming the consequent. It has already been mentioned in the last chapter when speaking of verification. The argument " If Jones were inattentive to his work he would go away for week ends " cannot lead us to the conclusion that he *is* inattentive *if* he does go away. There may be countless other reasons for his absence and he may not be inattentive at all. The frequency with which this fallacy

THOUGHT

is committed by employers and heads of institutions gives a poor idea of the logical powers of educated people.

FOR DISCUSSION

1.—Choose any outstanding question of the day. Read articles on it in the *Daily Herald, Daily Mail,* and *Morning Post,* and attempt to construct an unbiassed account of the matter.
2.—Devise and discuss means for training co-operative thought in schools.
3.—Consider the part which " association of ideas " plays in thought.
4.—How far is our power to reason correctly dependent on our general experience and knowledge, and how far on a " faculty of reasoning " ?
5.—What are the commonest fallacies we meet with in popular arguments—on politics, for example ? What teaching could be given in schools to warn children against such fallacies ?

BOOKS

Graham Wallas, *Our Social Heritage.* Esp. Ch. ii. This concerns the development of controlled thought.
A. Sidgwick, *Elementary Logic.*
Dibblee, *The Newspaper.* Home University Library. This book gives the facts about newspapers. The reader can easily draw his own conclusions about their impartiality.
S. Smith, *The Noodle's Oration.*
J. S. Mill, *Logic.*

CHAPTER XVIII

HABITS

" Absent thee from felicity awhile."

WILLIAM JAMES has maintained that we are creatures of habit and that a man is made or marred by the habits he forms. This is to some extent true, but the truth of the statement depends very largely on the number of activities which are included under the term " habits ". By strict definition those acts are habitual which are performed with little or no thought and always in approximately the same way. Such actions as doing our hair, dressing and undressing, or drying after a bath, are habitual in each one of us ; we give little thought to them while we do them, they are performed in approximately the same way on each occasion ; and, though this is not essential, they are matters of personal peculiarity. In all cases the habit has been formed as the result of repeating our actions, and the actions which we now do so easily were once the subject of anxious thought. As an example of a firmly established habit, we may take writing our own script. We learned to write with pain and difficulty, now our hand moves nearly as fast as our thoughts, and the mechanical difficulties of writing have almost ceased to exist. If we write in a script with which we are not so familiar, e.g., Greek, we give more thought to our writing. If we are copying a totally unfamiliar script, such as Sanskrit, all our attention is concentrated on the technical difficulties of the writing, because we have no *habit* of writing it. In common speech, however, " habit " is often used with a wider sense. We speak of " habits of tidiness and obedience " and also of "habits of thought". These are not really habits in the sense given above, and they will be discussed later.

Looking at the matter broadly, we can say that habits arise in the service of instincts when the conditions are sufficiently uniform. They are the line of development opposite to intelligence. Intelligence was said to be the power of adapting our behaviour to new circumstances, habits are the crystallized reactions when conditions remain constant. They thus serve a useful purpose in life. Where no thought is needed, they economize effort and set the higher mental processes free for other activity. Indeed, the performance of a habitual action has a soothing and stimulating effect. It is said that many a man's best ideas occur to him when he is shaving!

In the broader sense of the word also, habits economize effort. "Habits" of thought or feeling make us ready to respond in the required way without the necessity of thinking the matter out afresh, or imaging for ourselves the particular results of action. For example, most people, who are old enough to remember vividly the last war, have a set antipathy to war; and this antipathy is ready to flame up without fresh thought or consideration. They do not need to go through the old arguments about the wastefulness of war or its inconclusiveness; they do not need to call up in definite form the pictures of horror or the anguish of uncertainty, the word by itself sets off the sentiment which all these experiences have left, and the emotional reaction follows at once. This stabilizing of emotional reaction gives us our prejudices; it also gives us our principles.

Habits of the first class mentioned—true habits—are generally matters of skill, either physical or mental, and include such processes as walking, riding a bicycle, talking with a particular accent, repeating poetry and doing simple arithmetical calculations. These are all accomplishments which are acquired by repetition, and, when acquired, show the characteristics of true habits in that they demand little further thought.

A large part of school work is devoted to forming these habits, whether in the classroom or in the playing field, and it is necessary for the teacher to know something of the laws which govern the formation of such habits.

The simplest way of studying them experimentally is to learn for oneself some habit such as the following : On a piece of white card, about 12 inches square, mark a circle of dots, thus :

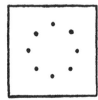 then, taking a pencil or a hat-pin in the *left* hand, and looking for guidance at a mirror, not at the hand itself, go round touching each dot exactly in the middle : A friend with a second hand to her watch —or better still, a racing stop-watch— takes the time for each attempt. If a curve of the results is plotted, it will be found to be of approximately this shape.[1]

Curve : results in groups of five.

A section of the curve showing variations in success at each attempt. Attempts 10–20.

Attempts 60–70.

These curves have been given in some detail because they illustrate some important points in connection with habit formation.

(i) The rate of improvement is not constant : improvement is much more rapid in the earlier stages of learning than in the later. Fig. 1 shows this. In the first *ten* attempts there is an improvement of five seconds ; another five seconds are gained in the next *twenty* attempts, and the remaining 40 attempts do not enable a saving of another five seconds to be effected. The same fact can be seen from the other two figures.

(ii) Progress is not constant, especially in the early stages. All attempts to keep up the standard of achievement are insufficient to prevent lapses such as those which occurred at trials 11, 19 or 68.

In the earlier series, the results fluctuate between 30 and 16 seconds ; in the later series the range covered is far less, and the worst and the best scores are 14 and 10 seconds respectively.

(iii) Besides these individual fluctuations, there occur

---

[1] Curves from writer's own experiments.

PROGRESS IN HABIT FORMATION

Attempts 10–20

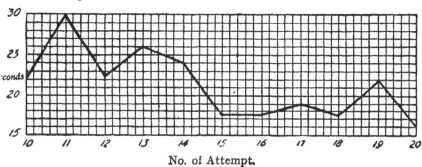

No. of Attempt.

Attempts 60–70

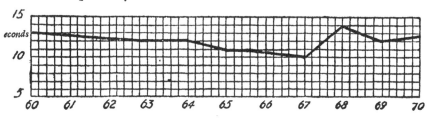

No. of Attempt.

Attempts 1–70, arranged in groups of 5

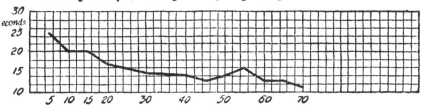

No. of Attempt.

flat places (even in Fig. 1), when general improvement seems to be at an end. Between attempts 45 and 60 in Fig. 1, there is little or no improvement, and in Fig. 3, from 60 to 66, there is a period during which the subject appeared to " stick ".

These three facts have educational bearings, and to grasp them may save the teacher much disappointment.

(i) When a new habit is being acquired, practice is extremely valuable, and the returns in improvement are high for the amount of time spent on it, but as the pupil improves, practice yields less and less improvement in proportion to the time employed.

Consequently there arrives a stage at which practice—as practice—ceases to be profitable ; where it is far better to take the practice incidentally as part of an activity with another purpose. To take two examples from school work : When a child is learning to write it is worth while concentrating attention on the writing and devoting periods to copying script, but as writing becomes easier, such periods do not produce any return proportionate to the time spent on them. Therefore it is better to let the children get incidental practice in writing in composition or other lessons. The second example concerns a habit which is more mental than physical—addition of figures. When a class starts to learn to add or subtract, practice in these processes is necessary, but when a certain skill has been acquired, it is better to go on to other rules and to allow the simpler processes to perfect themselves at the same time that new work is being done. Very few of us ever reach our maximum efficiency in simple arithmetic. The rapid improvement we make when we have, e.g., a set of examination marks to add and to reduce to percentages, shows how much might be achieved by constant practice—yet it is not worth while for the average person to give this practice.

(ii) The variations in efficiency which are such a conspicuous feature of the learning curve, often cause much heart-burning in school. They are recognized on the games field, where the player says he is " off his game " or " getting stale " ; but in the classroom a lapse from a previous success is generally regarded as an outbreak of original sin, or a sign of that complaint, the bugbear of conscientious teachers,

" slacking ". Of course, it is necessary for a teacher to guard against these evils, and to point out to a child his failures, but the teacher can bear in mind that such lapses are almost certain to occur, and that they should be no cause for discouragement.

(iii) The flat places, or plateaux as they are generally called, in the learning curve are more serious, from the teachers' point of view, than the lapses. They appear, from experimental work, to be almost universal in learning, and their causation is often obscure. But it is well known that there is at least one outstanding cause that will always produce such a check in improvement, or even a retrograde movement—and that is boredom. If a child who had previously been making good progress " sticks ", the teacher can look for various causes, e.g., health, home difficulties or diversions, but she must never neglect to ask herself if the child is finding sufficient scope and interest in his work. This problem is largely one of incentives. For a sufficient cause most children can surmount difficulties which have long proved unsurmountable ; unfortunately, a teacher is often not in a position to supply an adequate incentive. Most teachers use all their influence all the time, and when a special spurt is needed they have no extra or reserve power to draw upon, and, in consequence, they cannot give their pupils the extra fillip necessary to lift them over a difficulty. In cases of this kind it is frequently marvellous what effect a change of teacher will produce. The new stimulus applied in a new way or to a fresh spot may just make the difference which is required. This is one argument in favour of a class of children changing its teacher every year, rather than keeping the same teacher all through its school days as sometimes happens, especially in Continental countries.

There is one point which is not shown by the curves given but which is important in this type of learning, and which has already been referred to in the chapter on memory. Practice is most effective in forming this type of habit when it is spread out fairly thin. Short periods of practice should be given on successive days rather than longer periods on the same day. There are various reasons for this, the most prominent being that short periods do not produce fatigue and boredom and their greater frequency does not allow forgetting to occur in the intervals.

The aim in teaching habits of this kind is to make the activity so mechanical that it does not require conscious thought for its control. It is, therefore, essential to get the activity right from the beginning, because, if once a habit has been wrongly formed, and is then removed from the control of intelligence, the mistakes will be perpetuated. As is well known, a wrong habit can be formed just as easily as a right one, and once wrongly formed it may take months of hard work before the defect is remedied. Thus if once you have formed a habit of saying " th " for " s ", it is much harder to learn to pronounce the sound rightly *after* the wrong habit is formed, than it would have been to learn it correctly at first. The same thing is true of games. " Learn the right way *at first, start well,*" is the advice of all experienced players to beginners.

This fact is not always clearly realized in schools. If mistakes are to be avoided in the formation of habits, the early stages of habit formation must be watched over very carefully and every precaution taken to prevent a child from doing the thing wrongly. Too often a teacher gives a command and discovers afterwards that the class misunderstood what was expected of it. Or she spends much trouble in getting the class to form a habit which she later requires them to dismiss in favour of another. A curious point arises in connection with writing. It is customary now in many schools to teach script writing in the lower part of the school and insist on its being used ; in higher classes script is discouraged or forbidden, and a cursive hand desired. The teaching of script is said to have great advantages, especially in that it helps children to learn to read. If script writing be allowed to develop by degrees naturally into a cursive hand, the practice of teaching one habit and then changing to another would be psychologically unobjectionable. But in some schools any natural transition is forbidden until the moment decided upon by the head-teacher, when the children are required to drop script writing completely, and adopt a cursive hand. The change is so sudden that the writing-habit has to be begun again almost from the beginning, and much valuable time is wasted, and much undesirable criticism of school methods provoked from the more intelligent children. This is an extreme case, but something of the same sort frequently happens in arithmetic, when a class is taught one method of working a sum, made to practice it until it becomes habitual, and then is subsequently taught a "short method".

If a teacher decides that any activity is to become habitual she should make up her mind in the beginning what she wants, and give practice in that particular activity from the start.

The second and third types of habit are less easy to discuss since they are not or should not be true habits in the sense given above. Many of them are sentiments and have been discussed in an earlier chapter. In school many of these sentiments are cultivated under the name of "habits". We have "habits" of neatness, punctuality, obedience, courtesy, but in each case it is a *sentiment* not a habit which is formed. The actions which these "habits" lead to are not invariable but are adjusted to particular circumstances. On one occasion it may be polite to say "yes" and on another "no". It may be neat to stack books in a pile, to put shoes in a row, to put your hat on a peg and your stockings in a bag. If these virtues are merely habits they will not carry over from one case to another, nor, more important still, will they be proof against vicissitudes of fortune. Habits rapidly break down under excitement or when circumstances are greatly changed ; that is the reason why some of us suffer from stage fright and forget our part under the excitement of facing the audience, and why fear will make men do things which they would not do when calm. The vast disorganization of national life, which revolution and tyrannies bring, is not solely due to the material upheaval. The habits of the nation crumble away under stress of strong feeling and unprecedented circumstances. Therefore, punctuality, frugality, humanity, courtesy, which were merely habit, vanish. Men in fear of their lives, in circumstances which are strange, lose the habits which had previously guided them ; only those who possess real sentiments are able to retain their code of conduct. In the realm of morals, then, in so far as we have merely formed habits, our teaching is a partial failure ; a habit is better than nothing at all, but it is less useful than a sentiment.

The third type, habits of thought, would be better called " methods of thought ", and are due to sentiments and native tendencies combined. The finished product affords the best example of what is meant. A man who has received a training as an engineer is acutely conscious of the importance of accuracy and will rage at the incompetence of a drawing office which produces plans a tenth of an inch wrong. This love of accuracy will extend to other branches of thought, and such an one prefers to refuse all information on a subject rather than give a little without full and definite knowledge. The pursuit of other studies, especially litera-ture, does not conduce to the same accuracy of thought ; in fact, a certain extravagance in speculation is actually an advantage to a literary critic in these days, when all reason-able paths have been explored, and all likely hypotheses stated. This method of thought also tends to spread to the desire to make out a good case, and will frequently vanquish the desire to be strictly truthful. We can see how the different elements mentioned above enter into the produc-tion of the two types of thought ; native endowment largely determines the line of work adopted ; the actual pressure of daily work along certain lines forms a tendency ; admiration for great men of science, or bold speculators, forms a sentiment for the qualities which they obviously possessed.

In school we desire to cultivate certain of these methods of thought. We need to give children a conception of the value of accuracy, at least in certain matters, so that when they grow up we shall be able to trust them when they tell us our train goes at 8.15 p.m. We wish them to learn to verify statements or opinions before proceeding to definite action on the basis of them ; we wish them to have an operative belief in there being two sides to a question, and a tolerant attitude to the side which their neighbour prefers ; and we wish them to realize that " absolute truth " is a very slippery and changeable thing and that they are most un-likely to be in possession of it.

The task of the educator is not only to form habits but also to break them. Many children acquire bad habits in school, such as biting their nails ; or come to school possessed of them, such as a rough manner of speaking. The first necessity, of course, is for a person to be aware that he has a certain habit. Some people go through life with an exasperating sniff, or a curate's giggle, and never know that they possess these defects. We must, therefore, as a first step, point out to children the characteristics that we wish to change. It is, however, useless to indicate a fault unless we also evoke a desire in the child to amend it. This may be done by ridicule, but it can seldom be done by " nagging ". It can most often be done by appealing in some way to the child's other desires. People will not like the boy if he sniffs, the girl will spoil the look of her pretty hand if she bites her finger-nails ; if a child wishes to sing in the school concert he must learn to use his voice better, and not yell so as to roughen his notes. In other cases a habit has grown up under certain conditions and a change in circumstances will bring about a break in the habit. Where a habit persists long after the conditions which caused it have changed, it is probable that some obscure satisfaction is gained from the idea with which the habit is connected ; as, for example, when a man carries on certain habits from his days of prosperity into less fortunate times.

Closely connected with habit is the whole question of personal, as opposed to political conservatism. Some people are greatly disturbed by any change in their customary surroundings. If they go to church and fail to secure their usual seat, they feel that they have lost half the benefit of the service. A cook " always has " followed a certain menu, week in, week out, and is horrified at any suggestion of variation ; or the careful housewife " makes a point " of cleaning the silver on Wednesday, and cannot allow her custom to be disturbed for anyone's convenience.

This conservatism is a complicated thing. It springs partly from an identification of oneself with the activity, so that one feels a personal slight involved in the suggested alteration ; partly from a lack of energy to adapt oneself to new circumstances. Under the old conditions action could proceed with the minimum of thought, under the new conditions more thought is required, and to think means an effort that is felt as irksome. This state of personal conservatism is generally called " getting into a rut ", and is particularly common in later life when the total amount of energy at the person's disposal is less than in youth. It is a type of behaviour very difficult to deal with or remedy, since it is dependent on tendencies stronger than reason.

FOR DISCUSSION

1.—Rousseau recommends that we should " form a habit of forming no habits "—in order to avoid becoming the mere slave of mechanical action. Discuss the dangers of becoming " a creature of habit ", and suggest how these dangers may be avoided.

2.—Sketch the kind of way in which you would attempt to teach " a habit " of toleration of other's opinions—if you would teach it. If not, say why you would not do so.

3.—Try to account for the apparently useless habits some people develop, e.g., of twisting a waistcoat button when talking, of playing with a pencil while lecturing, of scratching the back of the head when thinking. How would you attempt to break any such habit which seemed undesirable ?

4.—Make a list, for your own edification, of activities which have become habitual to you. Which do you consider the most helpful in economizing time and effort ?

5.—Describe some habits which, when once formed, are hindered if thought is given to them, e.g., the habitual movement in riding a bicycle.

BOOKS

W. JAMES, *Talks to Teachers*, Ch. viii.
BAGLEY, *Educative Process*, Ch. vii.
JACK LONDON, *Call of the Wild*. The conflict between habit and nature in a dog.

CHAPTER XIX

INTELLIGENCE

The measure of this Universe.

THERE is a kind of mental efficiency, compounded of most of the elements that have been mentioned, which is commonly called *intelligence*. It is a quality very difficult to define, but very easy to recognize. It is the power to deal with situations as they arise, to learn and to think. One can see it clearly in a little child of two, and an experienced teacher maintains that she is hardly ever wrong in her estimate of a child's general mental efficiency. It is often measured roughly by a person's success in school examinations, or, where there is no certainty of equality of teaching, by a test which is supposed to indicate the general knowledge that a person has acquired. It is important to assess this intelligence because it gives some indication of the suitability of certain people for advanced instruction, or their capacity to learn and perform certain types of work.

The theory of the intelligence test illustrates what is assumed to be the nature of intelligence. Of the various powers of the mind as many as possible are tested. Often the power tested is only vaguely understood and the test is a rough-and-ready one. In one famous and widely used test the qualities chosen are simple arithmetical calculation, knowledge of language, comprehension of statements, power to follow directions, to apprehend analogies, and good memory.

This is a heterogeneous test and its chief merit is that it is wide. It shows not what a person can do in one specific field, but indicates roughly his abilities in many directions. If a person has powers of analysis, memory, skill in simple arithmetic, quickness, and so on, he is fairly certain to be able to do *something*. If, moreover, he has learnt the meaning of so many words or collected so much general knowledge he is likely to be able to learn more things in the future.

This type of test, on the whole, works well. It is definitely superior to an ordinary examination as a test for children, and when it has been applied to large numbers of adults for a special purpose the results have been good. It is worth considering the general theory rather more closely.

It is the ordinary custom to divide intellectual powers into two kinds : general intelligence and special abilities. The latter are quite simple to understand. A child is " good " at drawing, arithmetic or music. He has a special power in one of these directions and this power can be used without involving other powers of the same kind. Some children seem to have very few powers, others a considerable number, a few have ability in some one direction and a complete lack of it in all others. In a school or college it is quite interesting to pick out the special abilities of the

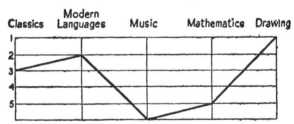

children, and if grades 1–5 are given for abilities in different subjects it is possible to make a graph of a person's abilities.

The above graph would represent a child quite good at languages, with no musical ear, poor at mathematics and really good at drawing. The average child is more con-

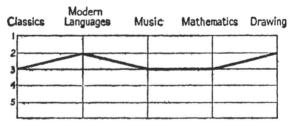

sistent. He generally achieves a fair performance in all subjects, though he may be better at some than others.

Such a child causes his teachers no anxiety. They know exactly what to expect from him, and his work is consistent. On the other hand, a child with outstanding ability in one subject, or with a complete inability in another, causes far more trouble. Teachers are always trying to explain away his anomalous brilliance or bully him into bringing his "weak subject" up to the level of his other work.

Far more difficult is the idea of "general intelligence". This is the general efficiency that the test was supposed to disclose, and we come back at once to the confused heap of powers that are too general in their use or too small to stand out as special integrated abilities. If we make an attempt to bring some order into this heap we can only do so tentatively.

In the first place there is the characteristic of general mental energy. It has been mentioned before. It is usually closely associated with physical energy and shows itself very early. To begin with, it is usually apparent as physical vigour. The small child who possesses it runs, jumps and is incessantly active. As the child gets older the more specific intellectual elements show themselves, and the child demands a succession of stories, toys, and, quite soon, to be taught to read and write. By three or four such a child is tired of the nursery and clamouring to be sent to school. If kept at home it gives way to bursts of temper, showing its indignation against a régime that denies it adequate opportunities for self-development. When it goes to school it is attentive, eager and very pleased with itself. Occasionally there is this vigour without many intellectual gifts. Then the child has to be provided with occupations or interests suitable to his abilities. Otherwise he is likely to become a "bad boy", and generally gets himself into the police court—if for nothing worse than for playing football in the streets.

The next and perhaps most universal is the power to grasp a situation. This involves direct apprehensions, and the power to organize the experience that is apprehended. A very good example was provided by a girl of two. Coming into the room at breakfast-time she looked round and said, "Uncle Roland, you haven't got your tie on." The uncle replied, "No, I know. I couldn't find it. I dropped it somewhere. See if you can find it." The child went away and came back with the tie.

The same child, when her brothers were wanting to play Punch and Judy, went off to the nursery and came back with a doll she thought suitable for the game. She even remembered, in the latter case, to take an adult with her to open the nursery door.

This grasp of a situation remains throughout life the chief character of intelligence. It depends on an organizing power of mind that varies very much from one individual to another, but which is present to some extent in all. It is also connected with memory. Certain types of memory—especially a parrot-like power of learning words—exist as a special talent and need not be associated with general intelligence. But many forms of memory are closely connected with intelligence. As was said in the chapter on memory understanding of the material and the possibility of organizing it as part of a larger whole are the most important aids to memory. It is just these qualities which are associated with intelligence. Furthermore it was said that memory was purposive, and could frequently be trusted to provide just the information that was needed at the moment. So here again organization and memory are connected.

The special gifts of memory, however, play no small part in earning a child the reputation for intelligence. Many of the school subjects, e.g., classics and modern languages, parts of history and geography, demand the power to learn words. A child who can do this easily has a great advantage over a child less well equipped and in many cases the appearance of intelligence is greatly increased. When we find a child learning poetry with great facility we regard him as intelligent. In this case there is both the power of verbal memory and the power of organization and understanding.

This capacity for ordering the experience we have is often made the central point of intelligence. Spearman [1] gives as two of his principles of cognition :

" Mentally presenting any two or more characters (simple or complex) tends to evoke immediately a knowing of relation between them."

[1] *Nature of Intelligence* and *Principles of Cognition.*

244

As an example he would give the learning of two musical tones and the apprehension that their relation is a fifth.

And " The presenting of any character together with any relation tends to evoke immediately a knowing of the correlative character ", e.g., if we hear one tone and think of a fifth the second tone suggests itself to our mind.

It is not possible to believe that musical appreciation is as fundamental as Spearman makes out, it only takes place when the English musical scale has been learned and understood. It does not hold for a very young child, nor would it hold, probably, for a Chinaman educated in the music of his country. The same thing is true with many of the wholes of which we learn to understand the relationships. The *particular* cases must often be the result of learning. What we do possess is the power, with experience, to apprehend their relationships.

This same central core of intelligence has been described in rather different terms but with fundamentally the same intention, as a state in which the specific response is modified in the light of the whole situation. Suppose an alley be constructed with wire netting at the bottom. Suppose a creature be placed at X and something desirable at A. If the creature at X be a hen it will continue fluttering

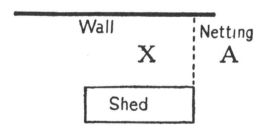

at the wire trying to get at A. If the creature is a dog it will make one or two efforts to pass the wire and, having failed, run round the shed. A child of 3 or 4 years looks about it and, understanding the position, goes round the shed at once. Here as in the other cases the important thing is the power to understand the whole situation and to adapt behaviour to the situation as understood. The same power can naturally be carried on into the intellectual sphere.

The relationship between this general intelligence and the

special abilities is that, on the whole, the greater the general intelligence the brighter will the special abilities appear. Even very brilliant special gifts in one direction will be little use without general intelligence, and general intelligence will often enable a person to do well in a subject for which he has only moderate special gifts.

From the point of view of general success there are other characteristics of importance besides intelligence. One is steadiness of purpose and persistence. People again differ very much in their possession of this quality. It shows itself in children mainly by the control of the attention. The abler child, as Mme. Montessori has remarked, plays longer with any occupation he takes, is quieter and more absorbed. The noisy, chattering, volatile child has probably less ability than his more absorbed neighbour. In adult life the quality is still important. The attention in all normal adults is far more stable than in children, but persistence, the power of sustained effort and the ability to endure disappointment are valuable qualities.

There is also a quality that has a high value in life that is not touched by any of the ordinary intelligence tests, and that is inventiveness. When the situation has been understood, then ideas should be ready to solve any problem that may arise. This has been discussed in the chapter on Thought, but its importance as part of intelligence cannot be overstressed. Every person who is in a position where problems cannot be settled by the application of routine solutions needs it. The executive who has a set of regulations to apply needs to understand the problem, but he does not need to do any invention. He looks up section ii subsection iv, decides that his case is covered by that rule, and acts accordingly. The position of the advertisement copywriter, the special feature editor of a newspaper, or an author is totally different. Even a gardener wondering how to dispose of slugs and snails and having considered the apparent indestructibility of the creatures, may be driven to devise some new form of destruction. The inventive man is one of society's greatest assets, though, of course, like all good things, he can at times appear a curse ; and the inventive child undoubtedly has a difficult side that those less gifted do not show.

INTELLIGENCE

FOR DISCUSSION

1.—Test your class with one of the standardized group tests, e.g. Otis tests and compare the I.Q.s thus attainted with your own estimates of the children's ability and the results of examinations.
2.—Describe the signs of intelligence in a small child that you know well.
3.—Consider the relation between special ability and general intelligence in the case of e.g. Latin and Music.
4.—Is there a unitary musical ability ? or is this ability itself composed of a number of small powers ? Apply the same type of analysis to other " abilities ".
5.—Compare the ordinary type of Examination with the Intelligence test.

BOOKS

G. L. THORNDIKE, *Educational Psychology*.
G. THOMSON, *Instinct, Intelligence and Character*.
C. BURT, *Handbook of Tests for Use in Schools*. Mental and scholastic tests ; a study in vocational guidance (Industrial Fatigue Research Board, Report No. 33).

PART III

THE CONDUCT OF MIND

CHAPTER XX

MORAL TRAINING

" Think of the gulf 'twixt them and me."

In the two earlier sections of this book we have sketched two
aspects of mental life. The first section, which dealt with
instincts and emotions, gave in outline the main impulses
which govern the life of man, and which suggest the ends
towards which he is impelled ; the second discussed what
may be called the intellectual tools which are used in the
pursuit of these ends. Memory, imagery, thought, may all
be used for their own sakes and be, in themselves, sources of
pleasure ; but their fundamental purpose is the assistance
they give in attaining the aims which are set by the instincts. If man were a solitary animal we might end the
description of the mind here, but he is not. He lives in a
society and in particular relations with that society, and is,
therefore, obliged to modify his natural tendencies and
desires to suit the conveniences of his neighbours. To take
a very obvious instance : It is natural for a hungry child
when sitting at table to clamour to be fed, or to snatch at the
most attractive portions. In a well-conducted family he
rapidly learns to wait his turn, or if he helps himself, to take
only a fair share of what is provided. In the earlier
chapters on instincts, particularly in that which dealt with
pugnacity, many of the modifications due to social pressure
were discussed. These modifications extend through every

department of life. Almost all we do we should do differently if we had received no training or a different one. The process of teaching a child to adjust himself to society is the fundamental work of education. All the book learning that we expect a child to acquire is a part of this adjustment. Our present-day civilization pre-supposes some knowledge of what books contain, since to live successfully we must have some conception of the remote in space and time. At other times, when conditions were different, inability to read or write did not prevent success. The illiterate Charlemagne became a great and successful ruler.

This training in social adjustment is spoken of in various ways. Sometimes the more external side is emphasized, and we say that a child is " taught manners " ; sometimes the mental side is emphasized, when the process is called " moral training ",. or a " training in character ". Both points of view are perhaps combined in the famous motto, " Manners maketh man ", where " manners " must be interpreted not merely as the outward form of courtesy, but as the inner culture and goodwill from which true manners spring.[1]

If we are to take our place in society we must not only control and modify our impulses so as to bring them into harmony with the needs of society, we must also work, and work in a way which is not possible or desirable, except in a community. Social life brings with it division of labour, and in consequence demands from us close attention to a single type of work. This increases efficiency, but it imposes a much greater strain on the worker than does the more varied life which involves different types of occupation. The farmer lives a more natural life than the city clerk and has more varied work which puts less mental strain on him. In consequence, nervous disorders are less common among farmers than in other classes of the community—though greater abundance of fresh air may not be without its influence in this case.

The second aspect, therefore, of the individual adjustment, which we have to make to society, is to learn to do with the minimum of strain the work which the community thrusts upon us. If we are to do the best work for society we must study our own powers and capabilities, and it is

[1] Cf. Spenser's *Faerie Queene*, Bk. VI.

not slackness to take those precautions which are necessary for securing our maximum efficiency. The second part of this section will consequently deal with a few questions of mental hygiene.

Before we begin to discuss the means of moral training it would be well to say a little about the aim we have in view, and the particularly complex problem that faces the teacher in the elementary school to-day.

We wish to bring a child into harmony with the society in which he lives, or, at least, into harmony with the best part of that society, and, in consequence, the aim of training changes from age to age, and is different in different countries at the same time. For example, an English girl of the professional class grows up expecting to earn her own living and must acquire habits of work and independence which will fit her to be a teacher or a doctor, or to take up any of the other professions open to her. She contemplates marriage as a 50 per cent. chance and, though she may desire it, does not allow it to occupy her thoughts too much, lest, if she fail to marry, she may suffer too acutely from disappointment. A Japanese girl on the other hand, except in rare cases, is not expected to fend for herself, she looks forward to a life of dependence and devoted service as a daughter or wife, and cultivates those arts of charm and submission which are necessary to one in such a state. Her accomplishments, her virtues, and her vices are consequently different from those of the contemporary English woman. The English girl of a hundred years ago was in much the same position as the Japanese girl of to-day, and the training she received was more like that of the Japanese than like that of the modern English woman.

The general history of morals shows changes of the same sort. In a slave-owning nation the moral code of the upper classes is essentially aristocratic. Greek ethic is a good example of this. Not only are the virtues which it discusses those of a cultured ruling class, but it naturally shows a strong intellectualist tendency, since the ideal person it wishes to fashion is always possessed of a certain level of intellectual attainments. While other religions stress faith and authority—as again is natural when they are thinking of uneducated people—Greek ethic emphasizes the *intel-*

lectual effort of the individual to discover the right course of action. The climax of this type of ethic is contained in Aristotle's famous description of the " Magnanimous Man ".

" The high-minded man is he who being really worthy of great things holds himself worthy of them—for high-mindedness involves greatness of scale, just as true beauty requires a large frame. There is some object which ought most especially to occupy him. We hold that to be the greatest of all goods which we attribute to the gods, and which is the chief aim of all great men and the recognized reward for the noblest exploits, and to this definition honour answers. When he meets with honour, and that from upright men, he will take pleasure in it, although his pleasure will not be excessive, inasmuch as he has obtained at the outside only what he merits if not perhaps less—for, for perfect virtue, adequate honour cannot be found. But honour given by the common herd he will hold in utter contempt, for it will be no measure of his deserts. . . .

" The high-minded man justly despises his neighbours, for his estimate is always right. The high-minded man is not fond of slight danger ; nor does he court danger as a whole, since there are few things which he holds in esteem ; but a great danger he will encounter and upon such an occasion is unsparing of his life, since he holds even life on certain terms to be dishonour. He also loves to confer a favour, but feels shame at receiving one ; for the former argues superiority, the latter inferiority. And so he hears with pleasure of the favours he has conferred, but of those which he has received with dislike. Towards those in high position and prosperity he bears himself with pride, but towards ordinary men with moderation ; for in the former case it is difficult to show superiority and to do so is a lordly matter ; whereas in the latter case it is easy—and to be haughty among the great is no proof of bad breeding, but haughtiness among the lowly is as base-born a thing as it is to make trial of great strength upon the weak. He regards truth rather than report, and in both speech and action he is open ; for he speaks boldly from contempt of others. Neither is he given to wonder, for there is nothing that he holds great. Nor does he bear malice, for high-mindedness does not show itself by long memory of past events, but rather by entire neglect of such things. About the necessaries of life, or about trifles of any sort, he is the last of all men to make complaints or requests ; for to do so argues over-zeal in such matters. The high-minded man, moreover, ought to move slowly, and his voice ought to be deep and his utterances deliberate ; for he who busies himself about a few things will not be given to haste, nor will he, who thinks nothing great, be of shrill, quick speech ; for a high-pitched voice and a hasty step come from these reasons." [1]

This ideal has always roused the fury of Christian commentators, and well it may, for nothing could be farther from the spirit of the Beatitudes or the Pauline ideal of " Charity ".—But Christianity had a different origin and was intended for a class of society different in all respects from that for which Aristotle wrote. Taking its rise in a subject nation, Christianity spread among the slaves of the empire and from them penetrated to their masters. It embodied in its earlier form morals which belonged as essentially to the lower classes as Aristotle's Magnanimous Man did to the upper. Aristotle could never have understood the way in which Christian legend loves to dwell on shepherds watching their sheep, nor shared the emotion expressed in Mary Coleridge's poem—

> Mother of God ! no lady thou ;
> Common woman of common earth,
> *Our Lady*, ladies call thee now ;
> But Christ was never of gentle birth ;
> A common man of common earth.
>
> Never a lady did he choose,
> Only a maiden of low degree,
> So humble she might not refuse
> The carpenter of Galilee :
> A daughter of the people she.
>
> And still for men to come she sings,
> Nor shall her singing pass away.
> " He hath filled the hungry with good things "—
> Oh, listen, lords and ladies gay !—
> " And the rich he hath sent empty away."

---

[1] *Aristotle's Ethics*, Bk. IV., Tr. Williams, p. 95, s. 99. For a far nobler ideal, one which would be almost universally acceptable, see Plato's Character of the Philosopher. Rep. Bk. VI., 485.

A large proportion of the avowed and earnest Christians never make any attempt to observe a large part of Christian morality. Such men as Gordon did not turn the other cheek, or practise meekness, or seek peace ! The Church *militant* has wisely adopted a large part of the ethic of the fighting man, and this ethic is the same, no matter whose battles are fought. To find this warrior morality in its purest form one must perhaps turn to Japan. There (in a country which has, to a large extent, officially adopted the pacific religion of Buddha) we find militarism and its accompanying virtues highly developed. The legends of the Daimios and their fellows abound with instances of great physical courage and endurance of pain, faithfulness to death, and valour and resource in war. The position of women is not high, as it rarely is in a country and age where warlike virtues are supreme, and attention is centred in the men. To this day the Japanese maintain the tradition of a comparative contempt for life, and consequently suicide is frequently a virtue.[1]

A totally different morality again is that of business. The classical exponent of these views is probably Smiles, and in his writing emphasis is laid chiefly on such virtues as industry, thrift and commercial honesty (to be distinguished from the rough, generous fair dealing of warriors or princes). A few quotations from his most famous book will, by their omissions no less than their emphasis, show his point of view. The date of this work is 1859.

Individual effort, not forms of government, determines national welfare. Indeed " it is every day becoming more clearly understood that the function of government is negative and restrictive, rather than positive and active, being resolvable principally into protection—protection of life, liberty and property "—on the other hand " British biography is studded over with illustrious examples of the power of self-help, of patient purpose, resolute working, and steadfast integrity, issuing in the formation of truly noble and manly characters." Men of all ranks have shown these powers and " have acquired prosperity by close industry, by constant work, and by keeping ever in view the great

---

[1] Cf. especially the institution of *Hara-kiri*.

principle of doing to others as you would be done by ". Eminent politicians have had the same power, and so have writers, and " success in these lines of action, as in all others, can only be achieved through industry, practice and study ", and in short " the conditions necessary to secure success are not at all extraordinary. They may, for the most part, be summed up in these two—common sense and perseverance." [1] This ethic of industry is a product of industrialism and its virtues are totally alien to Greek and early Christian writers, as also is the other cardinal virtue of the bourgeoisie, respectability. In hardly any century till the 19th is it possible to think of men or women being praised for such a quality, and its embodiment, Mrs. Grundy, first saw the light in a play of 1798.

As new virtues have grown up so some old ones have fallen into desuetude. Hospitality is no longer a cardinal virtue and a modern god would no longer travel round, as Odin and Zeus once did, testing it by unexpected visitations. Generosity to beggars would hardly be made the subject of an English morality play as it is of a Tibetan ; [2] nor do modern saints lick the sores of the poor or become the ferrymen of dangerous rivers.

In England to-day there is a curious mixture of moralities, and the schools, instead of educating a special class, as they have always done previously, are attempting to educate the nation as a whole. We have the morality of a governing class which is represented largely by the " public school tradition ". Here the virtues of loyalty, courage, initiative and willingness to accept responsibility and leadership are fostered. On the other hand a large section of the community has a business morality, and expects its employees to show the virtues of meekness and industry which fit their station.

The task for the public schools is fairly easy. They are mainly concerned with the governors ; the secondary

[1] Smiles, *Self-help*. Notice the emphasis on the reward to virtue—prosperity—especially in material things. " To succeed " is everything ! It is interesting to note that Smiles was a clerk in what is now the *Southern Railway*, and wrote his earlier books in office hours. They brought him money, and he retired to praise the virtues of an assiduity which he had not himself shown.

[2] Thrimecundan. *Three Tibetan plays.* Bacot and Wolf.

schools, in the main, possess the business ideals, and hard work and efficiency are their watchwords.[1] In the past elementary schools, too, knew their place, and produced docile boys and girls with just sufficient skill in their three R's to make them profitable employees. Now the position in the elementary schools is different. The children who pass out of them may be Prime Ministers, M.P.'s, chairmen of County Councils, directors of business houses, University professors, or pit hands. Which morality should the elementary schools teach, and for what type of life should they try to fit their children ?

The tendency is for the public school ideal to spread downwards. It has been adopted to a considerable extent by the secondary schools, and is beginning to spread to the elementary schools. Such games as football and hockey have become commoner in these schools and are used for the same purpose as in other schools, to improve the physique of the children and to teach them a certain amount of physical courage, team work, and individual responsibility. The prefect system is being introduced, and an attempt is being made to teach independence and the art of wise government of others.

This change in the tone of the morality taught in the elementary schools does not pass without comment ; and the business world, supported by certain sections of the daily press, clamours that our schools are giving the wrong sort of training, and that either we teach too much and, therefore, unfit the children for manual labour, or that we teach too little and, therefore, the schools are ineffective and should receive less public money. Teachers cannot ignore these complaints, but it is necessary to understand what lies behind them before they can be fairly answered. If in the elementary schools we fit the child for a higher standard of living than he previously knew, the child who leaves the elementary school to take up work in the lower ranks of industry will demand in time better conditions in his employment. Knowing the joy of well-occupied leisure, he will demand more leisure and more money to satisfy his needs, and longer holidays for travel. Whether or not this

[1] For the product of these schools some 20 years ago cf. H. G. Wells, *The Microscope Slip*.

is desirable is a question which each teacher must decide for himself, but the whole basis of teaching will be affected by the answer that is given.

Leaving each teacher to choose his own aim in teaching, we can say that " the training of character " is one way of describing this aspect of moral education. The type of character aimed at will, of course, depend on the aim of education, but whatever the type, many of the means to its achievement will be the same. The fundamental question is, what is " character " and to what extent can it be " trained " ?

We use the word, " character ", readily enough, but the thing which it signifies is difficult to describe or define. By character we generally mean a composite thing due partly to native endowment, partly to training. It has been defined as " a system of directed conative tendencies ".[1] Each word in this definition is important. The conative tendencies are instincts which are part of our innate endowment, their direction is determined partly innately, partly by social training. The organization of these tendencies into a system is largely the result of training working on tendencies of relatively different strength.

Of the innate elements which produce differences in character, the first is a difference in the total disposable mental energy. Some people, from their earliest childhood, desire vigorously and exert themselves energetically to attain their desires, others are unstable or apathetic. This quality of energy is to some extent connected with physical health. A person in good health has more mental energy to dispose of than one in poor health, but if great vigour of mind is given by nature, ill health very often fails to subdue it.[2]

The second innate cause for variations in character is the difference in the relative strength of the instincts. If some instincts are relatively strong they will colour the whole character in one way, while a preponderance of others will colour it in another. For example, the parental instinct, on the whole, leads to acts of gentleness and pity ; though,

[1] McDougall. *Outline of Psychology*, p. 417.
[2] Many of our great writers have been physical weaklings, e.g., Keats, Pope, R. L. Stevenson.

when its object is attacked, it may lead to rage. Yet this rage is altruistic in its aim and different from that which springs from wounded pride or from other egocentric instincts. A man in whom the impulse to fight is predominant will find a *casus belli* anywhere and will fight indiscriminately for a good cause or for none.[1] Self-assertion will drive a man to struggle for place and power, and will render him susceptible to slights to his dignity, and overbearing to his inferiors.

No hard and fast distinction of types can, of course, be made purely on the basis of some predominant instinct, because all other instincts enter into combination with and modify the dominant one. A combination of parental tenderness with instinctive self-assertiveness may give the type described by Bernard Shaw in *Getting Married*.

" Yes, my wife *was* a good mother ; such a good mother that all her children ran away from home " ; or the self-righteous person commemorated in the epitaph : " She had all the virtues—and her friends knew it."

The differences introduced by training are at least as important as those due to nature. These lie mainly in the direction which education gives to the instincts, and have been discussed earlier under the heading of sentiment. From the point of view of society it makes all the difference whether a man loves justice or horse-racing, whether he devotes his self-assertion to the field of public service, or to being an arch-swindler. Certain sentiments and certain innate tendencies are more or less incompatible—for example, the parental instinct if strongly developed would generally prevent a man from loving cruelty ; on the other hand a certain incongruity of sentiments is possible.

> When the enterprising burglar's not a-burgling,
> When the cut-throat isn't occupied in crime,
> He loves to hear the little brook a-gurgling,
> And listen to the merry village chime.
> When the coster's finished jumping on his mother
> He loves to lie a-basking in the sun.
> Oh, take one consideration with another !
> A policeman's lot is not a happy one ![2]

---

[1] Consider for example the alleged love of an Irishman for a fight. " Is this a private row ? " says Pat, " or can anybody join in ? "
[2] *Pirates of Penzance*, Gilbert.

It is in the direction of moulding sentiments that the bulk of the teacher's work in moral training is done. He chooses out those virtues which he wishes his pupils to acquire and sets to work to build up sentiments for these in the way that has been described.

Unfortunately the teacher is generally less influential in forming a child's character than the home environment. A child may believe what a teacher tells him, but he sees a pattern of life daily enacted before his eyes in the home. From his home environment he forms ideas of how people live, the right attitude of one member of the family to another, the relations of the family to the world outside. If the child belongs to a family where there is mutual love and forbearance, where the parents pay their debts, do their work and maintain pleasant relations with their neighbours, he is receiving a good moral training and is likely to show these virtues in his own life. If he grows up among criminals or semi-criminals and learns to regard all honest men as " mugs " and ordinary work as a want of a good intellect, it will be very difficult to alter these ideas. Once a child has formed his outlook on life he will have to suffer extreme vicissitudes before he will change it. Occasionally reformed criminals recount their life experience and we can see that a change of ideas is necessary before a change of life can take place, and usually this change is produced by a conviction that their ideas have failed. This conviction only arises when their activities have produced extremely unpleasant consequences, and it is here, if anywhere, that punishment finds its justification.

The parent or teacher has the task of giving a child its principles or prejudices. A child, on the whole, believes what it is told, especially if example and precept agree. If a child is consistently brought up to believe that such and such a course of action is right he will follow it, and these families acquire a tradition. There are families in all ranks of life in which the tradition of public service is strong, whether the service is done as check-weighman in a colliery village, local J.P., or Cabinet Minister. There are others in which all the members paint or play a musical instrument. This training of character is one of the most important sides of home life.

258

The organization of the whole character is not likely to take place within a child's school-days. As we grow older one set of sentiments acquires a dominant place in our lives and all the others fall into subsidiary positions around this. McDougall claims that only the self-regarding sentiment can bring about such an organization, but this does not seem strictly true. In some cases the dominating sentiment in a man's life is his scientific work, based perhaps on the instinct of curiosity. It is certain that the self-regarding sentiment becomes attached to any other sentiment that is dominant, so that we feel that we are realizing ourselves, and triumphing or failing through our work, but this does not mean that the self-regarding sentiment is the sole organizing force. The merit of a character, of course, depends on its dominant sentiment. The miser, dominated by his love of money and fear of insecurity, is socially undesirable, while the man whose guiding principle is a love of humanity may confer great benefit on the community.

The methods by which this adaptation of the individual to the environment is achieved, may be grouped together under the word " discipline " ; which has, therefore, a wide sense. It suggests both positive and negative values. It is positive, in that it attempts to form sentiments and sublimate instincts ; negative in so far as its aim is to repress certain manifestations of instincts which are socially undesirable. Unfortunately the positive side of discipline has too often been forgotten, and the negative side been thought of mainly in connection with punishment. It is a sad fact that it is almost impossible to train up a child " in the way it should go " without some resort to deterrents, and the simplest and most obvious of these is fear, caused by physical pain. The result is that such proverbs as " Spare the rod and spoil the child ", represent only too well the popular thought and practice of a short time ago. The unsatisfactoriness of fear as a means of controlling action has been discussed before. The modern educator is gradually learning to use other methods.

The whole question of punishments is an interesting one. To claim the right to punish implies a claim of superiority and right of jurisdiction agreed upon by a number of the community. But these claims are not always conceded by

the victim. A teacher may punish a child committed to his
charge, but if he attempted to punish a colleague, he would
run the risk of being sued for assault. In consequence the
proud are apt to resist the claim of anyone to " punish "
them ; and the idea of even divine " punishment " rouses
the anger of many. It is a different matter when unpleasant consequences follow an act, not as the result of
" punishment ", but as the " law of nature ". Then there
is no second personality involved and the pride of the sufferer
is not hurt. If a boy is caned by a teacher he may resent
the punishment extremely ; if when climbing a tree he slips
and falls, suffering thereby a much greater hurt than when
he was caned, he just takes it as inevitable, picks himself up,
and goes home to get his cuts washed. In the same way,
if we do something which makes a friend angry, and in his
anger he refuses to have anything more to do with us, and
leaves our letters unanswered, we are sorry and make
propitiatory offerings till his temper improves ; but if,
instead of giving way to nature, he remarks in a superior
fashion that to *punish* us he will not write for so long, we
probably decide that his attitude is intolerable and break
off the friendship ourselves.

The attempt, therefore, to represent natural results as a
punishment, especially as a divine punishment for our sins,
is a mistake. Nurses are fond of this attempt, so are those
who oppose certain medical reforms, maintaining that
disease is a punishment for " sin ". On the contrary, the
aim should be to make humanly instituted punishments,
where these are necessary, appear as like the natural consequences of an undesirable act as possible. If the retribution
is always the same, if it is no respecter of persons, the feeling
of personal tyranny is reduced and hence the resentment
felt by the victim is less. It is impossible always to allow
the child to learn by the strictly natural consequences of his
acts ; they are sometimes too serious, and the connection
between the act and its result is too obscure, but nothing
can replace experience as a teacher. With older children,
at least, the reasons for the law can be explained, and the
regulation be shown to depend on nature, not on caprice.

In schools the negative side of discipline is bound to bulk
largely. School education is an essentially unnatural

thing, and makes demands on the children which are completely at variance with their innate tendencies. For a human child, as for a kitten, a life of movement and exploration is natural. He needs to exercise his limbs ; to acquire knowledge of objects by touching and pulling. A small child running about a room, asking endless questions, is very like a kitten clambering over the chairs and creeping behind book-shelves. A kitten of about seven weeks old keeps his attention fixed on an occupation for about a minute, frequently less, the human child of five years or so is capable of longer periods of attention, but it, too, needs frequent change of occupation. We take these children, shut them up in buildings frequently stuffy and ugly to the last degree, place them in hard and uncomfortable desks, and ask them to remain still for long periods, while they give their attention to subjects which are in themselves of no natural interest. If the unfortunate pupils shuffle their feet, nudge their companions, talk or do any of the hundreds of things natural under the circumstances—they are called to order, because they are interrupting the lesson. Discipline under such circumstances *must* be largely negative. When one introduces more natural forms of work, when children are allowed to move about, to work in groups, to do things with their hands, or even when they are given more attractive books to read, half the burden of discipline disappears ; and the teacher can revert to his proper function, and cease to have to practice that of a drill sergeant as well. Negative discipline, imposed from without, and maintained by punishment, can never be more than a means to an end. The aim of the educator should be to dispense with this type as soon as possible.

In a state, there is always the repressive law to restrain those who have failed to form sentiments which are necessary for the good of society, but the majority of us keep quite clear of criminal acts ; we rarely even *wish* to do the things which the law forbids. We shrink from murder and despise theft. The educator's aim throughout should be to make his pupils *want* to do what is right and to be unwilling to do what is wrong, i.e. : " To feel pleasure and pain in the right things." Repressive discipline can never be anything but the first step in this direction. It may possibly make the child unwilling to do wrong—it can hardly make him anxious to do what is right.

There is a curious superstition abroad, even to-day, a legacy from Puritan morals—that the right, or duty, must be unpleasant. It is the primrose path, the broad easy highway, which leads to the everlasting bonfire, while the path to Heaven is set with stones and briars—" a strait and narrow way ". A little dialogue, once overheard, illustrates this point to perfection. The speakers were two women, both teachers, one some ten years younger than the other.

Young Woman : " I've just been playing golf. I always feel virtuous when I have done that."
Older Woman : " But you enjoy it, don't you ? "
Y.W. : " Yes."
O.W. : " Then how *can* you feel virtuous ? "

The two standpoints were poles asunder. The feeling of virtue sprang from the conviction that exercise in the open air is good for the health and temper, and is, therefore, desirable ; the older woman considered that, if one was enjoying oneself, there could be no virtue in the action (though, of course, there need be no vice). We can contrast with this attitude the doctrine contained in the *Fiddler of Dooney*.[1]

> For the good are always the merry,
> Save by an evil chance,
> And the merry love the fiddle,
> And the merry love to dance.
>
> And when the folk *there* [2] spy me,
> They will all come up to me,
> With " Here is the Fiddler of Dooney ! "
> And dance like a wave of the sea.

The latter attitude is the one which is most beneficial in education. How can we expect children to *want* to be good if virtue is always in mourning, flagellating herself with a whip of thorns ?

The same morality has left us another legacy closely connected with the previous one : i.e., the aim of moral training is a strong will, able to resist temptation, not a character so well adapted to its position that it does not feel

[1] By W. B. Yeats.   [2] Heaven.

temptation. To take a concrete example, it is contended that it is better to have a craving for strong drink and to resist it, than to feel no desire for alcohol. In fact, that it is better to be in a state of strain and distraction than to pursue a virtuous life, free from disturbances. Aristotle said that the sign of a formed moral habit was that the agent took pleasure in doing the things that were right, and that the man temperate by formed habit was superior to the man who was always struggling against temptations. A truly "good act" is one which proceeds from a good character, without, therefore, any sense of conflict. In this he was right, but it has needed all the psychological science of modern times to convince the devotees of suffering that it is so.

If we cannot learn to wish to do right always, the restraining force, to be satisfactory, must come from ourselves, not be thrust on us from without. Discipline must become self-discipline. This again, is only possible on the basis of formed sentiment, we must learn to love the virtues and hate the vices before we can criticize ourselves, or keep ourselves in the paths of virtue.

FOR DISCUSSION

1.—Sketch the main differences of method between education in a book-using community and in one which does not use books. Which modern methods are a reversion to an earlier type of teaching ?

2.—Sketch roughly and briefly the ways in which education has attempted to adapt children to the different types of morality current in Europe since the days of Themistocles. (At least Greek, Roman, Mediæval, landlord, and industrial eras should be touched on.)

3.—Give the chief dates in the history of elementary education, and indicate what important political events they closely follow. Show the connection between these events and the development of popular education.

4.—Make out a case to prove that the man who feels and resists temptations is better than the man who does not feel them.

5.—What do you think of the principle that you should never strike a child in anger ?

6.—Study the different methods adopted in schools for securing the co-operation of the children themselves in the work of discipline.

7.—Most religious communities see in discipline a training for the soul. Try to explain and discuss this point of view.

8.—What are the aims of military as distinct from educational discipline ? Should military discipline have a place in education ?

9.—Why do people maintain that experience of life is the best discipline ?

10.—In what ways—in work and play—can you allow children in school to learn from their own mistakes ?

11.—In what senses is it true that " Virtue is its own reward " ?

BOOKS

J. W. ADAMSON, *Short History of Education.*

P. MONROE, *Textbook in the History of Education.*

BIRCHENOUGH, *History of Elementary Education in England.*

M. E. SADLER (Editor), *Moral Instruction and Training in Schools.* Vol. I, United Kingdom ; vol. II, Foreign and Colonial.

WHITE and MACBEATH, *The Moral Self.* A modern statement of ethics from a somewhat psychological standpoint.

MRS. SHERWOOD, *The Fairchild Family.* Moral education a generation or so ago.

MARGARET KENNEDY, *The Constant Nymph.* Shows the contrast between formal and natural education.

For the Japanese Ethical Code :

LORD REDESDALE, *Tales of Old Japan.* Esp. the Appendix on Hara Kiri.

JOHN PARIS, *Kimono.* Modern Japan. The book is unfair by its omissions. Its facts are correct.

BRADBY, *The Chronicles of Dawnhope.* A skit on modern educational methods.

MARK BENNY, *Low Company.* The effects of bad home training.

JACK BLACK, *You Can't Win.* A thief and his reform.

CHAPTER XXI

DISORDERS OF ADJUSTMENT

" 'Twere good she were spoken with, for she may strew dangerous
conjectures in ill-breeding minds."

IF the process of directing instinctive tendencies into socially
useful channels is successful, it produces a normal person
who is free from those peculiarities of character which
might render him unfit for ordinary life ; but too often the
process is not completely successful, and in one way or
another failures of adjustment manifest themselves. There
are amongst us all manner of peculiar people, many of
whose peculiarities spring from mal-adapted instinctive
tendencies. There is the woman—anathema to health
visitors—who keeps an army of cats in one room ; there are
the victims of sick-headaches whom the doctor pronounces
to be suffering from nerves ; there is the stammerer ; and
there is the misogynist who lives by himself in the suburbs
and will not allow even a charwoman to enter his house.
These all represent failures of adaptation to the ordinary
conditions of life. In some cases this mal-adjustment is
even more serious and the conditions known as neuras-
thenia, hysteria, or " shell-shock " develop.

In the past, various fates have befallen these ill-adapted
people. For many centuries a strange old woman was in
danger of being burned as a witch,[1] a man who saw visions
might be regarded as a saint or as a servant of the devil ;[2]
those whose condition was more serious might be put into a
madhouse,[3] or told that they had the " vapours " or some
other " genteel disease ", according to their station in life.

[1] V., for example, *The Witch of Edmonton*, by Dekker.
[2] e.g., Malvolio in *Twelfth Night*.　　　[3] e.g., *Faustus*.

The modern science of psycho-analysis is an attempt to do for these people what education and their own efforts have failed to accomplish.

There are certain principles which underlie the practice of psycho-analysis and are of general importance.

(i) *That instincts are permanent.*—It has been contended by William James that many instincts are not permanent. He even gives it as a definite law that " many instincts ripen at a certain age and then fade away ". This is probably true of many that he enumerates, such as sucking,[1] or that insatiate curiosity common to all active young animals which leads them to investigate every object in their environment ; but it is not true of the more important instincts. If a child with a strong tendency to dominate fails to achieve his aim, this instinct does not die—it may, on the contrary, grow stronger and find outlets in some new way. The sex instinct, when repressed, sometimes determines a morbid interest in, and horror of sex matters.

(ii) *That memories can be repressed.*—A memory or an impulse is said to be repressed when it is pushed out of the normal thoughts of the person. This repression may be of two sorts. (*a*) A person may achieve it wittingly, as when a deliberate effort is made to forget, and change and distraction are sought : or when certain thoughts are stigmatized as evil and definitely avoided ; or (*b*) repression may be done unwittingly, as when some occurrence, important at the time, passes out of memory without any conscious effort on the part of the person who forgets. It is contended that, witting or unwitting, this process is purposive. We repress the unpleasant because unpleasant memories or ideas are alien to happiness and efficiency, and should therefore be eliminated. The ordinary introspective evidence for this is conflicting. It is common knowledge that when we look back on a past period, e.g., our time at college, it is mainly the pleasant events which stand out ; on the other hand many unpleasant events stick in our minds, do what we will to get rid of them. The fact seems to be that successful forgetting is nearly always unwitting. By taking thought

---

[1] This instinct is not always evanescent. It lasts on in some kittens long after they leave their mothers, and many quite big children suck their thumbs.

we may form new interests and new desires to take the place of those that are lost, but we do not actively *forget* our sorrow. When it does pass from mind it does so without effort on our part. Here, as in much else, success is the reward of tranquillity, not of strife.

It frequently happens that repression achieves its aim ; the petty troubles of daily life—our quarrels with this person or that, our exasperation with John or Mary—slip away from us, and our thoughts are not embittered by them. In other cases repression is *apparently* successful, in that tendencies or memories *seem* to disappear, but really it shews itself ultimately to be unsuccessful because the memories persist in a deeper stratum of the mind, and show their presence by disturbances of the ordinary adjustment to life.

(iii) *That instincts can receive a substitute satisfaction.*— The third principle explains this disturbance. Instincts can express themselves by modes of behaviour which are very different from their normal manifestations, and which have a value rather as *suggesting* the desired conduct than as being it. They are, in fact, symbols. It was pointed out earlier that the activities characteristic of an instinct could spread from its natural object to some other object of a similar sort : thus the tendency to care for a child leads people to care for and pet any small young animal, such as a puppy or a kitten. This is carried much farther in many cases, and various objects not obviously similar to the natural object of the tendency come to receive its manifestations. The tendency to dominate gives some of the most curious examples of this satisfaction of a tendency in unnatural ways. A child very early begins to show a tendency to try to attract notice and to want its own way. It is at a disadvantage among other people because it is so little and helpless, but it will scream or bang a spoon on the table, or do anything else that lies within its power to get what it desires. A normal child in a normal environment rapidly establishes a compromise between his powers and his wishes. He learns when circumstances and adults are too strong for him, and when by a manifestation of " temper " he can achieve his aim. He learns to satisfy his desire for leadership among companions of his own age or younger, and, if he desires absolute monarchy, to construct a day-dream realm of obedient subjects. He may carry his self-assertion into other paths, and determine to " master " some school subject or some profession. But the defective child, or one placed in an unfavourable environment is in a different position, and his reactions will be different, according to the particular difficulties against which he has to struggle. If the environment is unfavourable, if he is snubbed and " kept in his place ", if his reasonable requests are refused, and all healthy outlets for self-assertion checked, the child may become a dreamer, withdrawing into himself and enjoying there the triumphs that are denied him here, and making little or no attempt to struggle with his surroundings. Or he may become unmanageable, seizing every opportunity to assert himself regardless of the damage he does to himself or others. This state of things occurs on a national scale under bad governments.

The violence of a revolution is nearly always proportionate to the tyranny which has preceded it. It was not British good sense so much as the comparative mildness of the Stuart rule that made the English civil war so different from the French and Russian revolutions. In individual cases in the same way, the hottest-headed reformers generally have a tale of *personal* oppression to tell. Those whom society treats generously seldom wish to perform more than a minor operation on the body politic.

A child who is handicapped by nature is apt to proceed differently. He often finds that his very ailment is a means of making himself the centre of attention. Thus he tends to emphasize rather than to overcome it. This characteristic is sometimes asserted to be commoner among women than men, and in so far as the environment is unfavourable to women this is likely enough. A woman who is treated as an inferior because of her weakness may well employ the one weapon that is left her ; hence she emphasizes her weakness, and, in its name, keeps a household at her feet. This point comes out clearly if we compare the health of women as represented in the literatures of different types of society. In the Sagas, where the women stand on very nearly the same footing as the men, no woman faints, has a sick headache, or any other " feminine " complaint. If her husband's murderers come to the house, so far from screaming and running away, she comes out and speaks them fair, so that she may have a good look at them, and pass on their names and description to the unborn babe who she hopes will be its father's avenger.[1] In *Clarissa Harlowe* the heroine faints nearly every time she has an interview with her father, and frequently in the intervals between these interviews. Tight clothing is partly to blame in the latter case, but Queen Elizabeth wore stays of wood, and they were doubtless tight laced, and yet she only fainted when she wanted to impress the Spanish Ambassador or get her own way ! There are to-day a number of people who dominate their surroundings by the weapon of " weakness ", and they are probably as often men as women ; but while a woman's disorders are generally localized in her head (so that she has headaches), a man's are apt to be in his stomach (so that he has dyspepsia).

The desire to dominate may thus take any one of a number of forms. Not infrequently it is in part responsible for a stammer, and, where there is no organic defect, cure is easiest along the lines (a) of taking as little notice as possible of the defect ; (b) in seeking to remove the child's sense of inferiority and giving him normal outlets for self-assertion.

It is by no means always easy to discover what lies behind the substitute satisfaction of an impulse. A woman who lavishes excessive care and affection on lap-dogs, and turns the house upside down for their benefit, may be possessed of an abnormal amount of maternal tenderness, or of a desire to dominate others.

The difficulty of diagnosis is increased when particular emotional memories are the basis of the disturbance, because in such a case there is no general tendency to be invoked in explanation. Some people suffer from a dread of enclosed spaces and are wretched in a theatre or a tube train. It is often possible to show that such dread represents some emotional memory that has been unwittingly repressed ; [2] but such a memory would not be the same in any two people and, therefore, each individual case must be investigated personally. The difficulty is further increased

[1] Cf. the *Laxdaela Saga*.
[2] Rivers, *Instinct and the Unconscious*, p. 170.

by the fact that theory in this matter is uncertain and that the phenomena to be investigated do not present a clear-cut group. There is a continuous gradation, as it were, from those memories which are fully conscious, and influence our conduct in rational ways, to those memories which are completely repressed and which influence us in an irrational manner. When ironing, we are careful to use an adequate iron holder because we have memories of past experiences when we burnt our hand through using one which was too small. We dislike Mrs. X. because she resembles Mrs. Y., and Mrs. Y., on more than one occasion of which we hardly ever think, has been rude to us. A middle-aged lady known to the writers is always frightened and runs into a shop if a horse in her neighbourhood prances. The reason, though she has only once been heard to refer to the incident, and presumably hardly ever thinks of it, is that when she was a child, she was knocked down by a carriage and pair. Another woman had a horror of cats, and under treatment remembered a fact she had apparently previously quite forgotten, that in her childhood she had been terrified by a white kitten which had had a fit when she was playing with it.

The difficulty of discovering these memories or impulses has led to the development of a special technique, that of psycho-analysis, of which the two most outstanding features are the method of word association and the interpretation of dreams.

Word association is directed especially to the discovery of emotional memories—*complexes* as they are generally called in modern psychology—and depends on the fact that a rush of emotion will often impede a swift response to a stimulus. In its simplest form this method is as follows : The experimenter has a long list of words chosen so as to include different aspects of life (e.g., wind, love, stranger, blood, ceiling, merry, etc.), and a stop-watch. The subject, the person to be analysed, is seated comfortably in a chair. The analyst then calls out the words one by one and the subject replies with the first word which comes into his head. The experimenter takes the time between the calling of the stimulus word and the response. In some people certain words will give a very high reaction time, i.e., there is a long interval between the stimulus and the response, and these words the experimenter takes as being connected with some repressed emotional memory in the subject's mind. The next stage in the process is to attempt to find this memory, and that can only be done by the subject himself. The experimenter tells the subject to think of the chosen word, e.g., water, and say anything that comes up into his mind. A train of ideas will be started leading eventually to some memory—such as a boating accident or attempted suicide, which had to all appearance been forgotten. Even unemotional memories may be recovered in this way, and the device is not a bad one to use in certain lapses of memory. The working of this method is shown by the following example. A subject in a psychological experiment was asked to learn a list of symbols and then had a story read to her. About a month later she was asked, unexpectedly, to write out these symbols, and then the experimenter said, " You had a story read to you, didn't you ? " The subject denied it, having not the faintest recollection of any story. She was then told to give the first word which occurred to her in response to certain words. The first was " Hot ", and she answered " Cold " ; the second " Table ", and she answered " Chair ". The third was " Prince ", and to that she never gave an answer, for the whole story (which concerned a Prince) returned to her mind suddenly and overwhelmingly.

The method of word association, though useful, has been largely supplanted by dream interpretation or analysis. One might try many words and not hit on one which would touch off the repressed memory ; but it is contended that dreams always have reference to the deeper thoughts and desires of the dreamer, and, therefore, are a more suitable starting ground. They also reveal more ; for they throw much more light on the general tendency of the subject's thought than does the word association method. Some dreams demonstrably refer to the wishes of the dreamer, and often these wishes are very little disguised in the dream. Many children, and some adults, dream of eating beautiful cakes—only in some, but not all, cases, this dream is spoiled because the cakes are tasteless. The slum child very often dreams of playing in green fields. Dr. Kimmins, in his study, *Children's Dreams*, notes that 28–42 per cent. of the dreams he collected from children of 8–14 years were wish fulfilments, and that among children in Industrial Schools, where the conditions of life were less natural, wish fulfilment dreams were half the number collected.   With adults this direct expression of wishes in dreams is rarer, though it persists with curious vividness in some cases.   The authors of this book had, through a mishap, lost their ruck-sacks on a walking tour.   The sacks contained all the necessaries of life for them for the next week.   It was not unnatural, therefore, that one of the owners dreamt twice in one night that the ruck-sacks had been found, and eventually dreamed also of a plan for their recovery.   Other dreams express the sleeper's desire less directly.   The following is a dream of a young teacher who disliked work and was hoping to get a post in a university or training college.

" I was out for a walk with the school, and we came to a hill.   I began to climb, and it was very steep, so that I had to use my hands to hang on with.   I had no shoes on, and felt the stringy stalks of heather between my toes.   The school straggled out a long way behind.   At last I got to the top, which was flat, and I was alone."   As in all dreams, the dreamer—or someone who knows him extremely well— is the best interpreter.   In this case the dreamer, yielding himself to any ideas which happened to come into his mind, lay thinking this dream over.   Almost the first association which occurred was the advertisement of a well-known correspondence college, which runs, " There is plenty of room on top."   This, taken in conjunction with the dreamer's circumstances, made the wish behind the dream clear at once.

On the other hand, dreams do not always represent a simple wish.   They more often represent a complex state of mind in which there is a conflict between a desire and circumstances, or one set of desires and another.   For example : A young man was staying in the country with friends whose main occupation was playing tennis, and he felt himself growing rather contemptuous of their way of life.   One night he dreamed that he had stolen the library copy of the *Life of St. Teresa*, and when accused of the theft was filled with confusion and made a lame defence.

The associations with the dream were immediate. St. Teresa at once suggested a picture of St. Catherine that he had recently bought, and that picture, with its air of superiority, suggested the line, " I don't look properly down my nose." The dream was felt to be a comment on his attitude to his hosts. He was " looking down his nose " at their amusements, and he had no right to do so—any more than he had any right to the library copy of the book.

Adults generally only dream of topics which involve some kind of conflict—if there is no conflict, if wishes are fulfilled, and action is straightforward, it is unlikely that a person will dream of these things. Dreams are a kind of sleeping thought, and like waking thought generally concern a problem. The reason why dreams have not been recognized as a form of thought is that the processes used in them are distinctly different from those that occur in ordinary waking thought. Yet it is well known that solutions to waking problems often occur in dreams.[1]

In waking thought the situation is often treated abstractly, and different solutions " argued out " ; in dreams both the problem and this solution are represented concretely in visual and dramatic form. This dramatic form gives the dream its peculiar character ; we really seem to be taking part in the events, not merely thinking about them, and the exigencies of this dramatic form influence the way in which ideas are presented. For example, a question may be represented in the dream as an attempt to discover the answer, and if the answer is not known the attempt may fail. On one occasion a brother was anxious to find out whom his sister had met on a certain day. He had hinted this wish but got no satisfaction. Next night he dreamt that she had received a letter from Z (whom he believed she had met) and that he was trying to see the post-mark on the envelope, because, from that, he would be able to surmise whether Z had been passing through Bedford on that day or not. The post-mark was illegible. This dream gave in a dramatic form the question, " Was Z in Bedford, because, if he has been, it is almost certain my sister met him ? " and it gave, also in dramatic form, the answer, " I don't know."

[1] Cf. Myers' *Human Personality and its Survival of Bodily Death*, App. ii.

To achieve these situations the dream uses many of the devices of the dramatist. If in a play an author wishes to show that a man is mean and avaricious, a scene is introduced to show him engaged in some money transaction, so that the abstract quality may be represented by some concrete instance. So in a dream a problem as to the whereabouts of a person is represented concretely by an attempt to read the post-mark on his letter. The concrete symbols used are often highly personal and depend on certain pieces of knowledge or reading. In a certain recorded dream the dreamer dreamt that she was killing a big dog. The explanation of this dream lay in a line of poetry that she had recently read :

" And soul, the stag, escaped the hound, desire," and was a dramatic representation of an attempt to bring a certain passion to an end.

In a similar way both dreams and plays involve various types of concentration. To put a complicated story into the form of a play, or to get an elaborate situation into the dream, many elements must be combined. The dramatist telescopes place and time, and the dream does the same even with people, so that it is no uncommon thing to hear a dreamer relate how he met someone who was his Uncle John, and yet at the same time was also his father.

These elements in the dream make it difficult, without study both of the individual and of dreams in general, to tell what it is that a dream signifies, and the true meaning is often to be arrived at only by following the chain of association back through more than one step. On one occasion, a woman anxious to put certain desires out of her mind, dreamt as follows :

" I was standing on a hill making a speech, and waving my arms and getting excited. . . ."

When asked for associations the first one she gave was college debates, where she used to speak (she had been down from college two years or more), and when asked which debates in particular, she replied, " One on prohibition," and asked for associations with that, she gave " Temperance ", which, in a wide sense, was the object of her thoughts.

A teacher, as a teacher, can have little direct concern with the interpretation of dreams. A normal child's dream can be safely ignored, and in abnormal cases an analysis generally needs more time and skill than the teacher has to give ; but occasionally a hint can be obtained from a child's dreams as to his needs, which might not be so easily obtained in other ways. It is not a bad plan to ask the exceptionally naughty child what he dreams about, and if his dreams show certain unmistakable wishes, to make enquiries into his home life along those lines.

The physician, however, who deals with the definitely abnormal, bases his treatment on the results of dream analysis. When he has found out the cause of the patient's symptoms he tries to remove it. If the patient is suffering from the repression of some tendency, he advises a way of life that will give this tendency more scope ; if the cause of the mischief is some emotional memory which is excluded from ordinary consciousness, he attempts to reinstate this, and so allow the patient to regard it reasonably and calmly. In many cases the mere facing of an unpleasant memory will deprive it of its power to harm.

FOR DISCUSSION

1.—Discuss the rise to power of Hitler from the point of view of its probable psychological causation.
2.—Write out any dream you dream frequently and compare it with your day-dreams. Can you suggest any interpretation ?
3.—Some poets, e.g., De la Mare and Coleridge, have an unusual ability in suggesting a dream atmosphere. Study their poems carefully, e.g., *Arabia*, *The Listeners* (De la Mare), *Kubla Khan* (Coleridge), and say what elements in these poems are dreamlike.
4.—Why do you think some dreams appear so important and others not ?
5.—Could you suggest any psychological explanation of the abnormalities of the character of Richard III, of the sleepwalking of Lady Macbeth, or of King Lear's madness ? (Refer to Shakespeare's plays.)

BOOKS

BERNARD HART, *The Psychology of Insanity*. A clear account of modern theories of repression and complexes.
C. BURT, [1]*The Young Delinquent*. A study of the means of dealing with juvenile crime, and in particular an account of psychoanalytic work in this field.

---

[1] For more advanced students.

W. H. R. RIVERS, [1]*Instinct and the Unconscious; Conflict and Dream; Psychology and Politics.* Essay III.
>Rivers was in charge of shell-shock patients during the war. He was also deeply interested in ethnology.

NICOLL, *Dream Psychology.* All the experts disagree about the interpretation of dreams. Note the differences between the books quoted.

JUNG, [1]*Studies in Word Association;* [1]*The Psychology of the Unconscious.*

FREUD, [1]*Interpretation of Dreams.*

ADLER, [1]*Individual Psychology.* Esp. Ch. i.
>These last four books are all long and difficult. They are *only* suitable for advanced students who intend to specialize in the subject.

MRS. HODGSON BURNETT, *The Secret Garden.* A charming children's book which anticipates most of the modern theories of education.

---

[1] For more advanced students.

CHAPTER XXII

MIND AND WORK

" I am not lean enough to be thought a good scholar."

THE previous chapter naturally suggests a view of the nature of mind different from that popularly held. We have spoken of memories being repressed, and, though apparently forgotten, still influencing our conduct. If we regard the mind as a unity, such statements are naturally hard to understand. Psycho-analysts, therefore, adopt a hypothesis of the nature of mind which explains the phenomena presented to them. This view is not only important in itself, but also has certain bearings on the conduct of our ordinary lives.

The natural view of the mind, based on common sense, and fortified by language and religion, is to regard each person as having a mind or soul which is a unity and conscious of itself. Now, though this seems so obvious, it is as much an hypothesis as any other view, and it is by no means universally held. Egyptian religion gave to man more than one soul ; many races believe that a man's soul—or some part of his soul—can be taken away from him by a magician and imprisoned, e.g., in a bamboo cane. Philosophers have declared the soul to have parts, Aristotle dividing it definitely into three, the vegetative soul (that concerned with the body), the appetitive and the speculative. Plato also divides the soul, but differently. We need not, therefore, feel that we are flying in the face of the opinion of the world when we distinguish parts in the soul and raise a doubt as to its unity.

The body of each individual passes through a long course of ante-natal development before it attains human form, and there is no reason to believe that the soul or the mind [1] does not also change and develop. In the first place, the control of the body, whether of the developing embryo, or of the adult, is a mystery. It is possible to give the facts in terms of physiology ; but, even so, the problem is stated rather than solved.

What guides the growth of the embryo so that, in spite of chances—of experiments even, the typical form of the creature is evolved ? There is no complete answer to this. The management of the body in adult life is hardly less marvellous. The presence of germs in the body will normally bring about an increase of white corpuscles in the blood, and the duty of these corpuscles is to destroy germs. Frequently the person in question hardly knows that his system has been so invaded ; he almost certainly does not know where and how the white corpuscles are produced. He may not even know that they *are* produced, yet his ignorance or knowledge makes no difference to the effective working of this very delicate adjustment. A similar case is the secreting of adrenalin during anger, fear, or pain. This secretion is followed by changes in the body favourable to great exertion, but disadvantageous when that is not needed. Even if we know that the secretion is going to take place, no thinking of ours will stop it. The examination candidate, who does not want his breakfast, cannot get up an appetite by any exhortation of his glands to stop secreting.

In the past it was argued that our body was a beautiful machine so perfect that it not only ran, but repaired itself, and looked out for jolts on the road. Now scientists are abandoning that hypothesis, and the more eminent the scientist the more completely he seems to have abandoned it. The theory was, indeed, the product of partial ignorance. When physiology knew less of the phenomena it studied, a mechanical interpretation was fairly easy ; now that knowledge is greater, and wonder after wonder, fine adaptation after fine adaptation is revealed, it becomes ever more necessary to postulate some power beyond the machine.

---

[1] Mind and soul are here both used of the non-material lively principle in man. There is no specifically *religious* connotation given to the one word, or *intellectual* to the other.

It seems almost inevitable to return to Aristotle's thinking, and to postulate if not a separate soul, at least some function of the mind which is concerned with the conduct of the body and is wise beyond the best physiologist. This part of the mind, in man, is withdrawn from consciousness. It is strange how abruptly our direct knowledge of our own bodies ends. We can know the external form of our hand, for example ; but if we want to know how it is that we move our fingers, we must look it up in a text-book or get someone else to tell us. We cannot discover the facts from our own bodies by any examination—physical or mental—possible to ourselves. We know if we have a pain, but often enough we do not know exactly where that pain is or what is causing it. A prick we can locate, but colic spreads vague but acute discomfort over large regions of the body. The ordinary person knows far more about the chair, which he sees, than about his own eyes, with which he sees it. Our very brain, in which apparently the mind resides, is unknown to us till we study it as an external object—generally as a lifeless one.[1]

We are so used to this condition of things that we do not marvel at it, yet it is one of the strangest facts in our experience. On the other hand, we marvel at those comparatively rare cases in which a mind takes direct cognizance of the states of its own body. Such cases occur occasionally, the most frequent being when a man has premonitions of death and knows that a certain sickness will be his last. A few cases are on record in which the patient was able to give accounts, varying in precision according to his degree of medical knowledge, of the state of different organs, and thus to guide the doctor's diagnosis.[2] In these cases there seems to be the recovery of a lost power rather than the development of a new one. Certain Hindus are said to be able to control their heart beats and the circulation of their blood.

It is easy to understand why, in the course of development, conscious thought ceased to be concerned with the bodily functions. If such processes as digestion needed

---

[1] The child is so unconscious of the workings of his body, that he frequently thinks of himself as a hollow tube in which he stores food.

[2] Osty, *Super-normal Faculties in Man.*

conscious thought before they could be successfully accomplished, we should have our minds occupied for an hour and a half after every meal. Only because such processes have been removed from conscious control can we find time for other thoughts. On the whole, therefore (whatever may happen in a particular case), this severance of the bodily functions from our conscious thought has been beneficial.

The attempt to divide the mind farther is more speculative,[1] but all the evidence goes to show that even our thinking is not done in a uniform way. We have commented before on the way in which dreams represent our thoughts and wishes, and in some cases solve our problems for us. But the processes by which they do it are removed from our consciousness. Dreams present us with the result of this thinking, but we are not able to watch the process as we can in ordinary conscious thought.

Another example, less common indeed, but for that reason the more striking, is afforded by post-hypnotic suggestion. A hypnotist can give suggestions to a good subject, which the subject carries out quite accurately after he has returned to normal consciousness ; although, having forgotten what happened to him under hypnosis, he is ignorant of the reasons for his act. Some of the most famous experiments on this point have taken the following form. A man hypnotizes a subject and tells her to make a cross on a piece of paper, and write the time of doing so, after 799 minutes have passed. He at once wakes the subject, who shows no sign whatever of remembering any of the events which occurred during hypnosis. She is sent about her ordinary business, but returns later with a piece of paper with a cross and the time of day on it. If asked why she has written it and brought it, she declares that she does not know, but felt impelled to do so. This experiment is interesting from several points of view : (1) It shows how motives of which we are not conscious influence our actions, resulting in feelings of impulsion which appear irresistible, even if unreasonable ; (2) if the subject is to carry out the

---

[1] This is one of the most interesting and confused provinces of psychology. For some of the literature on it, see the list of books at the end of this chapter. There are some questions on those books, but they are only for more advanced students.

command at the *right* time—and she does this—she must either count the minutes as they pass, or she must find out by calculation when the right time falls. In either case, whether she counts or calculates, this is performed without *conscious* thought. The experiment can be varied and the subject told to perform another task. On one occasion an unpoetical undergraduate was asked for a poem. He wrote one, a very bad one, and produced it blushingly, quite unable to explain his sudden deviation into verse.

A similar thing can be demonstrated with a crystal or glass of water. If a suitable subject be made to sit and gaze at one or the other, he will generally see pictures in it. The experiment is easy to do, and a fairly large proportion of people can see these " visions ". The water or the crystal should stand on something dark, and the light should be behind the subject's head, not opposite his eyes. These " visions " are practically waking dreams, and can be interpreted in much the same way as night dreams. The only thing to be careful about is that occasionally the experiment is too successful ; the subject passes into a state of light hypnosis. In that case it is better to stop at once. The psychological interest of the experiment lies in interpreting the " visions ", and discovering the mental processes which have been involved in their production, and which yet have lain outside the subject's conscious thought.

The terms used to describe the part of the mind which performs these unwitting acts are various ; we shall call it the sub-conscious, meaning simply by this that it is not conscious in the ordinary way. We can connect it with those emotional memories and unadapted impulses which we discussed in the last chapter.

The relation of the sub-conscious to the conscious thought, whose processes we can observe, is something like the relationship of a sea to the tidal estuary that is observed from the parade. The sub-conscious seems to be larger, more passionate, both more primitive and wiser than the conscious. Conscious thought is a specialized power intended for our dealings with the external world. It is a tool of marvellous complexity and fineness, but little more than a tool. The completeness of our limitation to conscious thought is a measure of our isolation and individuality. Conscious thought works through the senses and, it seems, through the senses alone. Even in internal thought, it employs images of one 'sort or another ; and when the sub-conscious wishes to communicate with the conscious mind, as in dreams, it does so by means of visual and other images, giving to its abstract meaning a sensuous form.

Conscious mind is the recipient of that training in continuous directed thought which was discussed earlier, and it is conscious thought which forgets the unnecessary and unpleasant, and acts as a sieve through which only relevant impressions can pass.

If once we realize this difference between the conscious and the sub-conscious mind, and that our personal limitations are mainly characteristics of the former, much that seems mysterious can be understood as part of a general scheme. There is little doubt, for example, that telepathy (i.e., direct communication between minds without the intervention of any ordinary means of sense) is possible. It is not possible for all of us, but there is quite sufficient evidence to show that it is possible in a great many cases. Intelligent research is beginning to show the conditions which are necessary, and it is growing clear that telepathy is closely connected with a certain general power, which some people have, of making the sub-conscious accessible to consciousness. The first condition of telepathy is a partial suspension of conscious thought, sometimes so complete as to produce a " trance ", sometimes only reaching a state of abstraction. In this condition images, often visual or auditory, sometimes emotional, present themselves. In as far as these images are *representations* of a more or less abstract fact, they may be hard of interpretation, e.g., death may be represented by a skeleton, an open grave, or an abyss opening at one's feet. Hence the language of seers is one of metaphors.[1] " I see . . ." and the hearer or the sage proceeds to interpret the vision.[2] The marvel of the proceedings (waiving those rare cases when something *absolutely* unknown is disclosed) lies in there being no ordinary means by which the seer could know the events disclosed ; but if it be realized that the sub-conscious can

[1] See the prophecies in the Old Testament for example.
[2] Osty, op. cit.

cognize facts in the minds of other people, without the intervention of sense material, then the marvel is only one case of a general principle—strange, but human.

The importance of this view of mind, theoretic as it is, lies in the possibility of applying it to conduct. If we are to do the maximum amount of work with the least strain we must study the mechanism and needs of the mind, just as a prudent motorist studies the needs of his car.

There is a certain tendency among earnest people to regard thought expended on mental hygiene as so much indication of slackness and tendency to hypochondria. It is not so, any more than the owner can be accused of pampering his car when he oils it. The man who rests wisely does much better work than the man who goes " all out " all the time ; and nowhere is this more obvious than in teaching. One could quote Scripture—" By their *fruits* ye shall know them,"—not by the fuss they make in getting their fruits in.

The problem before most workers is to discover a method of work which will allow them to accomplish what society demands of them without a disabling effort.

Modern methods of work and training put a strain on that fine instrument, conscious thought, which it is ill-adapted to bear, and if care is not taken of it the tool may give way. The problem, therefore, is two-fold : (i) how to get some of our work done by some part of the mind other than conscious thought ; and (ii) how to give conscious thought adequate rest. Both are essentially problems of organization, and if we find ourselves in a position where no amount of organization will relieve the strain, for our own sakes, and for the good of society, we had better " quit " and get another job.

(i) As has been said above, the conscious mind is the most convenient instrument we possess for thought, because it is the only instrument whose working can be controlled. It is the only means of getting through a job which requires to be done at once. Sub-conscious thought is less trustworthy, more erratic, and must be left to take its own time. Therefore, if we wish to employ this type of thought, we must make arrangements different from those which we normally employ. In particular we must be well in advance. It frequently happens to us that we have more than one piece of work to do ; that we have to write two lectures, one on English, one on psychology, and that we wish to finish a chapter of a book, all within the next day or two. There are two ways of facing the situation. One is to start on the English lecture and work doggedly at it, biting our pen when ideas fail, and staying up late at night reading books of criticism, in the hope that they may suggest something. When at last the work is done, we transfer our jaded minds to the psychology and follow the same course. The certainty is that the chapter of the book will not be written, and the probability is that the lectures, though full of matter, will possess no coherent ideas, and be worthy and dull. All the work has been done by conscious thought and, as it were, on a single line. It is possible, however, to use the sub-conscious to a large extent, and do much of the work concurrently. If, instead of starting straight off on one piece of work and leaving the other two jobs completely alone, we look at all three of them and decide what must be done about each, a large part of the work for the other two will be accomplished while the first is actually being carried out. Then, if the work is to be spread over two days (it is rather different when one spell of work is in question), it is generally more *economical* to start with the easiest piece of work ; then, while we are writing the comparatively simple psychology lecture, ideas on the more difficult English one are taking shape, and, when we do come to deal with it, we find that what before was agitated blankness, has become illuminated by certain fairly clear principles. In the same way it is a mistake for the busy worker to sit searching for an idea. Only novelists with private fortunes can afford to spend a whole day seeking the perfect word. Most of us cannot enjoy such luxuries. We need not abandon the word, but we must fill up the period of waiting for it to suggest itself by some other occupation than that of pen-nibbling. If ideas run out, we can consign the problem to the sub-conscious, and get on with some easier task till that mechanism produces the solution ; and, if we are working at a subject within our power, it generally will produce the solution in reasonable time.

It is even possible to leave the job completely to the sub-conscious and never consciously revise its work. Some speakers have great courage in this way. They know in advance that they must address a meeting on some topic. They know the kind of thing required, and think of it in odd moments, but go into the room with no definite notes of what they are going to say, and the speech is ready for them as they say it. Many teachers give their best lessons with only this amount of preparation, and not a few lecturers are most fluent and inspiring under these circumstances. Such a gift can be abused, but the most carefully prepared lecture is better if sub-conscious thought has been expended on it ; and, obviously, to get the bulk of one task done concurrently with some other is an enormous saving in time and energy. If we are to have a life outside our official duties, we teachers need to practice every economy of effort, and an intelligent anticipation of our intellectual needs is of the greatest assistance to ourselves and benefit to our work.

(ii) The second problem, that of using our conscious thought to the maximum without producing exhaustion, is a question of fatigue. Fatigue in physical work has received of recent years a large amount of attention, because of the industrial importance of the question. Speaking generally, we can describe fatigue in physical work as a decrease in power to perform work, the decrease being due to previous work ; and if fatigue is long continued, the whole efficiency of the person is so lowered that grave industrial waste is caused. Roughly, the output curves for a day's work are as follows :

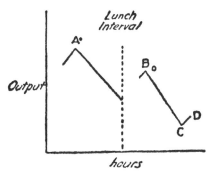

The points of interest are A, which shows the increase of

efficiency which comes from " warming up " to the job ; B, the increase of output after the lunch interval and rest, the warming-up period then is short ; C, the rapid drop at the end of the afternoon, and D, the final spurt as the hope of release grows. Investigations into the details of fatigue have resulted in various other discoveries, three of which are important here.

(1) Frequent short rest periods will postpone the onset of complete fatigue for a long time ; each rest period is followed by a rise such as that shown after the lunch interval.

(2) Increasing the hours of work beyond a certain point means an actual absolute diminution in output, because a state of chronic fatigue is established which depresses the whole standard of production. During the war, the shifts in the munition factories were cut down from twelve to ten hours and from ten to eight hours, and each cut was followed by an increase in total production.

(3) Fatigue (judged by the length of time necessary to recover from it) does not increase in a simple proportion, but in a compound. If a task A is done when fresh and produces fatigue of amount X, then the same task done when the doer is already fatigued produces a much greater amount of fatigue XY. This is a matter of the utmost importance and it should be considered whenever we are working " against time ". It is more economical to get up at 6.30, and do an hour's work before breakfast, than it is to do the same task late at night when we are tired ; and this for three reasons (a) the fatigue produced is greater when it is done at night ; (b) it will take us longer when we are already tired ; and if it takes one hour in the morning it will almost certainly take two at night ; (c) it will be better done in the morning. Work done late at night is almost always full of mistakes.

These findings with regard to physical fatigue are largely applicable to mental work—especially on its more mechanical side, but the exact weight to be given to each consideration depends on the constitution of the person. It is nearly always a mistake to work when tired, and the person who wishes to be efficient and healthy should make every effort to arrange his day with adequate rest pauses. Teachers at school too often ignore this, and fill up the lunch interval with the strident bustle of school dinner, or the pleasanter tasks of folk dancing or netball. Then, having taken home in the evening many books to correct, they take fright and sit down immediately after tea, before they have recovered from teaching, and dash at the pile. Later, perhaps with a headache, they sit up late preparing lessons —martyrs to their own lack of sense. Every school that has the welfare of its staff at heart should provide a really *quiet* staff room with comfortable chairs for use in the dinner interval : the afternoon teaching would improve out of all belief, if everyone had half an hour's sleep between the morning and afternoon school.

The problem for the individual worker trying to do the maximum amount of work is the best relation between rest pauses and the warming-up period. Some folk are badly disturbed by even a small interruption ; others can go away, drink a cup of coffee and come back without having lost the thread of the sentence at which they were working. Again, creative work differs from mechanical work in this, that ideas occasionally insist on occurring late at night, and to go to bed on those occasions at 10.30 (as health demands), would be to lose the most brilliant idea which had occurred for a week. Nevertheless, such nights of inspiration should be rare. They nearly always have to be paid for by a day of absolute stupidity afterwards, and once in three weeks or so is the limit of a wise man's indulgence.

However carefully we arrange our work some definite relaxation is essential. The most complete relaxation is sleep, which completely interrupts conscious mental activity, though it does not always interrupt that of the sub-conscious. The amount of sleep, which people need, varies from person to person, but most adults need to go to bed at about 10.30 p.m. and sleep until 7.30 a.m.

Sleep like most other things is affected by habit. There are people who allow themselves to believe that it is useless for them to go to bed before midnight, as they can never sleep earlier. In most cases this is merely a habit fortified by auto-suggestion. There is no reason, except their own belief in the impossibility of sleep, why they should stay awake, and no normal methods of inducing sleep succeed with them, because the real cause of wakefulness, their own belief, is unchanged. These people are generally suffering from want of sleep and find it hard to rise in the mornings. They are not those who by constitution need comparatively little sleep. If a person is *truly* unable to sleep the case is one for medical advice in order to avert a nervous breakdown. Sleep is, in fact, the great safeguard, and as long as a person can sleep well there is little danger of a serious breakdown. When sleep becomes broken, or very difficult, the case should be dealt with professionally.

On the whole those people need most sleep who are most nervously excitable when awake. The man of sturdy constitution and steady nerves can thrive on less sleep than the more excitable man. The misfortune is that a person with a nervous temperament is more liable to suggest insomnia to himself and thus lose the sleep which is especially necessary for his sanity and health. The excitable man, too, is frequently more active during his waking hours than the other. There are people who can sit idle and resting for an hour together, or prolong tea-time chat till six o'clock. Others are perpetually occupied all their waking hours, and never talk without sewing, or sit without a serious book. The more active person naturally requires more sleep to compensate for the hours which the other spends in comparative tranquillity. A desire to sleep and a great capacity for doing so is not, therefore, necessarily the mark of an indolent character ; on the contrary, it is frequently associated with great mental vigour. Not a few of the world's greatest generals have had it. Hannibal, as a young man, would drop asleep anywhere—according to Livy—and was always either asleep or working.

Sleep and work, however, should not occupy our whole lives. It is bad for us, because it diminishes our power ; it is bad for those with whom we come into contact, because it decreases the interest of our personality. Among teachers especially, a width of interest and activity is essential if they are to keep their freshness and hence the respect of their pupils.

Apart from this, relaxations are a necessity for mental hygiene. It has been said before that conscious directed thought is not a primitive function, and that it cannot be sustained even over all our waking hours. We need certain activities of a simpler type, which keep us happy and occupied, without putting a strain on those particular powers which are involved in thought. The great majority of men find such relaxation in some form of sport. Cricket, football, golf or tennis takes a large place in their lives. These activities are physically healthy and mentally recreative. Other men take to gardening. Such occupations can be carried out by the use of mental mechanism earlier in development than those required for work of an intellectual nature. Other recreations depend on various types of gregariousness, tea parties, concerts, bazaars, dances and what not. In yet other cases the recreations are definitely intellectual and are pursued by people with considerable powers of intellectual work, or by those whose ordinary occupations are inferior to their capacity. Thus the professor plays chess, works mathematical puzzles, or has lessons in Russian ; and the clever coal-miner goes to evening classes in literature.

The old saying, " a change of work is as good as a rest ", is partially true. The difficulty lies in deciding how *much* change is necessary. For the school child the change from Latin to Greek is less of a change than that from Latin to mathematics—school subjects which demand rather different powers—while a change to woodwork is far more of a change than either. So with the adult. An hour's hard digging in the garden may bring vast refreshment to the city clerk, but probably would not do so to the ploughman.

A change in emotional attitude has as beneficial an effect as a change of occupation. Our work too often fails to give us an outlet for our emotions ; our hobbies, in that they are felt to be expressions of our own individuality and power, satisfy us in a way that work does not. A very small change of occupation joined with this change in emotional attitude will bring great relief. It is one thing to write letters on the firm's business, quite another to write them on one's own ; and a teacher, who is wearied with explaining and arranging facts for presentation to a class, may turn with joy to just such explanations and arrangements of facts if he is writing a paper for a scientific journal.

The refreshment which this change gives, renders it very necessary for the worker to have friends and interests outside his work and the institution to which he belongs. If one's friends are employed in the same institution, the emotional atmosphere is too constant. School or office gossip tends to intrude, and " shop " is always on the edge of the conversation. Get a friend who does not care, and probably does not even know about the problem of Molly Jones' scholarship or John Smith's bad manners, and the whole atmosphere is different. The problems can be forgotten, or even made the subject of a joke ; the sultry atmosphere of *Mr. Perrin and Mr. Traill* [1] can all be blown away by one good laugh from a cynical outsider. Those of us who have lived among people obsessed by the little worries of school life know how irresistibly comic the whole thing appears when related to someone who moves in a different sphere. The laughter we provoke by our tales of woe at first hurts our vanity, then we feel the outside point of view and laugh too, and the danger is past.

This matter of adequate relaxation demands thought from most people who are taking up posts for the first time. It is so easy to believe that work will and should be all sufficient, and to hope that amusements and friends will present themselves unsought. In too many cases they do not, and the institution gets a firm grip of the individual and starts sucking his blood like a vampire ; only to throw the victim aside twenty years later, completely worn out.

Men on the whole are more fortunately situated than women. A larger proportion are married, and if home life after business hours brings added cares, it also brings relaxation in a change of duties and conditions. The unmarried woman needs to think carefully and to choose some line of relaxation for herself. It may be church work, art, sport, or politics, but definite planning and effort are necessary if she is to provide herself with a life of her own, and such relaxation as will enable her to carry on her other work to the best of her ability.

This relaxation of the adult can be interestingly compared with the play of children. There is a very great apparent contrast. The adult slips back to a lower level, " becomes a boy again ", the child is striving upward, imitating his elders and trying over in advance his future activities.

[1] Hugh Walpole.

290

A six years' darling of a pigmy size
See where 'mid work of his own hand he lies.
See, at his feet, some little plan or chart,
Some fragment from his dream of human life,
Shaped by himself with newly-learned art ;
    A wedding or a festival,
    A mourning or a funeral :
    And this has now his heart,
    And unto this he frames his song :
    Then will he fit his tongue
To dialogues of business, love or strife ;
    But it will not be long
    Ere this be thrown aside,
    And with new joy and pride
The little actor cons another part;
Filling from time to time his " humorous stage "
With all the persons down to palsied Age,
That Life brings with her in her equipage ;
    As if his whole vocation
    Were endless imitation.[1]

Attention has often been focussed too exclusively on this aspect of children's play and theories have been put forward which have suggested that play is a preparation for life ; or, since children often imitate antiquated adult activities, such as hunting with a bow and arrow, play has been explained as a recapitulation of the life history of the race. It is true that children are imitative, but the imitation arises in a desire to try to use his growing powers rather than from any occult impulse to recapitulation. It is also true that through play children acquire skill for future actions ; but this skill could be acquired as well or better by work. The fact is, that it is the nature of healthy living things to be active, and for a child to be inactive is usually a sign that he is ill ; but to be active one must do *something*, and a child does what he is able to do, which is activity of a simple type. He runs and jumps, whittles sticks, makes mud pies. These activities correspond to certain ancient tendencies in him and take certain forms through the traditions which come down to him. The child who knows of knights-errant goes off with his sword of lath to slay dragons—another who has never heard of such tales takes a very similar sword to slay a policeman. As each new power develops it appears as a play activity till it is caught, brought under the control

[1] Wordsworth, *Ode on the Intimations of Immortality.*

of steady purpose and attention, and made to work. Since such control of thought is the latest and most unstable of our acquisitions, the adult is always slipping back to the play of the child and adopting his simple physical actions and enjoying spells of child-like spontaneous attention.

FOR DISCUSSION

1.—What are the religious difficulties raised by " multiple personalities " ? Have you any solution to offer ? If so, what ?

2.—[1]In what ways can we distinguish the conscious, co-conscious and unconscious ?

3.—[1]In what ways is the word subconscious used in psychological literature ? What do you consider the justification for each use ?

4.—To what extent is the school time-table arranged with reference to the principles (a) of variety, (b) of fatigue ? Give concrete examples.

5.—Study the day of an average teacher and indicate in what ways the arrangement of work could be improved ?

6.—Give various theories of play and say what facts support each and which you personally believe.

7.—Study the play of a kitten over a period of one or two months and note the different forms it takes.

BOOKS

MORTON PRINCE, *The Dissociation of a Personality*. One of the most amazing of scientific records ; [1]*The Unconscious*.

F. H. W. MYERS, *Human Personality and its Survival of Bodily Death*. Esp. App. II.

F. C. S. SCHILLER, [1]*Doris Fischer Case of Multiple Personality* (proceedings of Psychical Research Society, Part LXXII, Vol. xxix).

GROOS, *The Play of Man*. The theory that play is a preparation for life.

WILLIAM JAMES, " The Gospel of Relaxation ", in *Talks to Teachers*.

W. McDOUGALL, *Body and Mind*.

---

[1] For advanced students.

CHAPTER XXIII

HAPPINESS

" In a contemplative fashion, and a tranquil frame of mind,
Free from every kind of passion, some solution let us find."

THE adjustment of our intellectual powers to the demands of life is, if anything, less important than the adjustment of our emotions to these same demands. Successful work is an ingredient in happiness, but success need not bring happiness. It is on the emotional side of our nature, and on the richness and rightness of its relation to the circumstances of our life that happiness mainly depends.

The ideal life would be one in which all our tendencies received an harmonious gratification. This is not to say that we should live a life in which every whim was gratified, or one in which we abandoned ourselves to every passing emotion. Our own natures are too complicated to allow of that. To gratify one impulse is often to baulk another more important, and the earliest lessons in self-control aim at showing a child that, for his *own sake*, he must compare the ultimate gratification to be derived from different courses of action, and choose that which on the *whole* brings the most pleasure. The adult has continually to face the same kind of problem, and, to take the lowest view of the situation, he must, from purely selfish considerations, curb the expression of passing emotions, and study the happiness of others in an effort to gain his own. A life, therefore, which affords us gratification for our various tendencies is not a life of impulse or selfishness. Owing to our gregarious nature and our need to give and receive affection, a life which satisfies most of our desires may be one of self-restraint and devotion. There are many charming families

293

in which one is struck at once by the air of happiness which pervades them. The members of the family are contented, they have about them the things they desire, and they are engaged in occupations which they like. Yet their satisfaction of desires has not meant the gratification of selfish impulse. A happily married woman with children and a sufficient income is another example of the same kind. She is engaged in looking after her house and family, in paying social calls, and takes part in local politics and the affairs of her church or chapel. Her life is a satisfaction of her natural tendencies, and yet it is not selfish or lacking in restraint or regulation.

Unfortunately all folk do not achieve such a harmony between their tendencies and their position in the world. Most of us have to face certain mal-adjustments which may be due to ourselves or to our surroundings or circumstances. There are men and women who are never happy anywhere, there are others who could be happy and would be so if their circumstances were different. The people who are incapable of happiness have already been discussed. They are fit subjects for psycho-analytic treatment. The others, who form a large proportion of mankind, are able to fight their own battles and attempt to solve their own problems. Roughly, these problems fall into two groups : the control of the manifestations of temporary emotions, and the control of those circumstances which lend a permanent emotional colouring to life. The first is the more obvious problem and, therefore, may be taken first.

We have said before that much of the early training of a child is directed to giving him a control over the manifestation of his emotions. On the general principle that restraint is bad, it is far better for a child to feel a desired emotion than to repress an undesired one ; but no amount of training will enable the ordinary person to pass through life feeling only such emotions as are convenient. An unexpected accident will terrify us ; a slight, perhaps unintentional, will fill us with jealousy ; or a failure plunge us into despair.

In regard to emotions people are differently constituted. There are some of very stable emotional make-up who are little moved by the chances of daily life. They are the reasonable men, who do not take offence, or get excited or worried, who love calmly and deeply, and act after due thought. They do not fall victims to the wiles of an Iago and they make, perhaps, the best schoolmasters. They are trustworthy ; their calm comes not from stupidity and insensitiveness, but from an innate balance and stability. Their opposites are of the hair-trigger variety, off at a touch and sorely the victims of their own excitability. They spend much of their lives struggling against bursts of emotion which their reason condemns as unjustifiable ; and, unless they do so struggle, their bursts of passion, gaiety, or despair will unfit them for a place in society as at present constituted. A third type feels perhaps more deeply than either of the other two, but does not react in the sudden manner of the second type. Whereas the extremely excitable person is apt to be incapacitated by his own rush of emotions, speechless with anger or sobbing with grief, this third type is rendered more efficient by the first stimulus of emotion, but the emotion makes itself felt later and, when the moment for action is past, takes possession of his being and haunts his dreams and casts a shadow on his life.

The calm type has few problems to face ; the explosives, if they wish to get along in fair tranquillity, need to study themselves and their surroundings, and avoid causes for emotion rather than stifle it when it has been aroused. There are certain situations which always rouse Jones to fury ; and if he is a wise man he will go out of his way to avoid them.[1]

It is often possible to catch a burst of anger brewing, and by a definite course of thought to check it. For example, a plan is on foot for a picnic. We feel that we are the person best qualified to give advice about the locality. But our opinion is not asked ; in all discussions we are ignored. Our pride is hurt, we feel our temper wearing thin. There may be only one safe course of action, to lose interest in the plan altogether. So long as we allow ourselves to think about it, there is the continued irritation of the implied insult, but if we can persuade ourselves that the picnic is for us the least important thing in the world, that we are really too busy with other matters to desire any part in it, and so forth, though indeed " the lady doth protest too much " for real

[1] V. Spenser, *Faerie Queene*, Book II., Canto iii.

295

conviction, yet an outburst is avoided, and, in retrospect, we shall be so pleased at our intelligence in keeping our temper, that we may almost forget the discourtesy of the other party. A few emotions can be stood up to and argued down, but it is often better to run away and play the ostrich, than risk the exhaustion and degradation of an undesirable display of uncontrolled emotion.

The problem for the third type is more difficult still. A certain amount of emotion is a temporary advantage, and it is hard to judge the violence of the after effect. There is a tendency to let oneself go for the sake of the eloquence or the vigour that emotion gives, and to hope that after all the future may not be as bad as last time ; but, when the full force of the emotion comes, the circumstances which produced it are past. There is no outlet and little sympathy available, and turned in on itself the flood does more damage than when expended naturally on an object. A confessor or a confidant is perhaps the best hope for such as these, and a little talk and friendly chaff will often console and relieve.

As in all else it is well worth while to be honest with oneself over emotions, and to study one's own mental make-up, discover one's *bêtes noires*, and take reasonable precautions. There are so many events and chances in life that cannot be guarded against, that it is reasonable prudence to foresee and avoid those strains and stresses which can be anticipated.

This is the negative side of emotional control ; the positive side is if anything more important. In the chapter on sentiments some of the methods used by society in producing the emotion that it desires have been discussed, but this process has its effect without the individual making any personal effort and generally without his being conscious of the process. It is frequently necessary for us to take our own part in this, and to develop for ourselves the sentiments of which we stand in need. Society sees to it that we become fairly honest and industrious. It is the graces and amusements of life that we must cultivate for ourselves, since without them, though we may be efficient, we are not likely to be happy. Roughly, language includes these sentiments under two heads, " taking an interest " in certain things and " forming friendships ". The one group of sentiments fits us for solitary life, the other for social, and both are essential to happiness, since man must have objects of various sorts on which to expend himself. There is no state more miserable than the blank boredom of having nothing to which to turn our attention, or no friend who needs our care.

It is one of our first duties towards our mental health to supply ourselves with abundant and suitable interests, and that is not difficult. The world is full of cheap and innocent amusements—botany, sketching, artistic crafts, bee-keeping, horticulture, amateur dramatics and bridge. We can study music or literature or become photographers. We cannot stand alone naked to the world, and any of these subjects will act as a cloak.

It is possible to live solely on things, but it is far better to find one's solace with one's fellow-men. Many hobbies naturally lead to pleasant associations. One joins a society and attends meetings, and takes tea afterwards ; and thus one finds human objects to receive one's affection and interest. But unless these acquaintances ripen into friends the full benefit is not gained. A friendship does not spring up like a mushroom in the night, at least not after one's first year at college. It is an edifice that requires careful rearing, it is founded on confidence and admiration, and is built of common experience and mutual service. A good friendship is the highest work of art, and like all the noblest creations is the product of joint effort. In a friendship one has that restrained freedom of action that was mentioned at the beginning of the chapter, and of all the constituents of happiness none is more important than a good friend.

In consequence we should seek friends, and, having found them, give thought and care to the relationship. Very few friendships are such sturdy plants that they need no care. We must watch both our own actions and those of our friends. We must study the effect of certain situations, and try to bring about the pleasant ones and avoid those which are likely to breed dissension or pain. This sometimes limits our action. We may like long walks ; our friend may be a confirmed potterer. It is better to avoid a walking tour altogether than to quarrel on one. In a similar way we may sometimes forgo the pleasure of a meeting rather than go and find our friend so immersed in the rehearsals for a play that he is unable to take any notice of us and so hurts our feelings. As was said above, happiness lies in an honesty that allows us to anticipate events and choose those most productive of general well-being.

Just as the individual must exert himself to achieve happiness, so society is beginning to take account of man's individual peculiarities, and in an attempt to secure efficiency, is really making for happiness. Most people are better at some one thing than others ; they are more efficient if they work at this, and they are generally happier. Square pegs in round holes do not bring profit to themselves or others, and in consequence science is being called in to supplement the rough chances of ordinary arrangements.

The present system depends partly on accident, partly on the idea which each man forms of himself. We have discussed in a previous chapter the formation of the self-regarding sentiment, and it was shown that this sentiment always includes an idea of oneself as possessing certain characteristics and capacities. As we are likely to order our life in accordance with this idea, it is of no little importance to form a correct estimate of ourselves. In the ordinary way we are helped to do it by " knocking about " among our fellow-men. The boy at school learns his place in work and games ; the student fails or passes in his examination, and takes a leading or minor part in college affairs ; and the man is reprimanded or praised for his work.

This verdict is generally accepted, too generally, perhaps ; but it not infrequently happens that a man who is a failure as a teacher feels sure he would be a good journalist, or an unsuccessful tram-driver secretly longs to be a house-decorator.

A more exact method of evaluating capacity than we possess at present is desirable both for the happiness of the individual and for the advantage of society. This valuation may take two forms : a general test of a general quality called " Intelligence ", or a test for specific qualifications, such as those involved in, e.g., salesmanship or typing. Intelligence tests are of direct use in education as a means of grading children and placing those of approximately the same powers in the same class.[1] It is also of use in other fields. During the war all the recruits for the American army were tested, and those of superior intelligence selected for special training as officers. The results were said to be very satisfactory. In civil life the same thing applies. It requires a higher level of intelligence to be an engineer than a stoker, and it is wasteful and dangerous to put too good a man at a poor job, just as it is dangerous to give a fool responsibility.

The work of scientific testing is as yet in its infancy, but at some future date we may hope for a general grading of the population which will allow the more naturally intelligent, whatever their wealth, to get into superior positions, and the less intelligent, whatever their parentage, to fill the humbler.

The other branch of the subject offers infinite scope, and only the outside edges have been explored. At present various factors co-operate to determine the choice of a profession. Taste is occasionally consulted, but more often other considerations are paramount, such as the cost of the necessary education, family convenience (such as having an uncle in the business), locality, or just mere chance. Of the hundreds of young men and women who start teaching on leaving college, only a small proportion would adopt that profession if all the world were open to them on the same terms. The comparative ease of entry and the fair security of position tempt them to lay aside their natural inclinations.

The first essential, in an ideal state, is to consult the inclinations of individuals as to their occupation. A person may be bad at almost every kind of work except the one for which he feels himself fitted, and this type of work he will do well, to his own pleasure and the public profit. A small example shows the type of thing meant. A certain large London store had an assistant who proved incompetent in one department after another ; at last, when they were on the point of dismissing her, the welfare worker asked what she *wanted* to do. " Oh," said the girl, " I've always longed to be among flowers." There was a floral depart-

---

[1] The literature on this subject is very large and continually increasing. At *least* the books given at the end of the chapter should be read.

ment to the store, and the girl was tried there. Her success was immediate.

In this case the girl's idea of herself corresponded to the reality. In the majority of cases this is so. If we really *want* to do a thing we can generally achieve a certain measure of success in it, if only because of the trouble and thought we are willing to expend on it. Occasionally we are mistaken about our own capacities. There are also people who have no preferences, and regard all ways of life as " work " and nothing more. For both these classes of people some external guidance is necessary, and at the present time investigations are being carried out with the aim of devising tests which will indicate fitness for special occupations. The most successful work, perhaps, is being carried out in connection with flying. There are certain qualities of steadiness and quickness which are essential for a pilot, and tests have been invented and have met with considerable success in the selection of those who wish to be civilian pilots. The whole problem is necessarily very extensive, especially in the case of industry, because in one factory there may be hundreds of different processes all requiring different aptitudes. Yet a very fair start has been made, and when the utility of the task, both to individuals and society, has been grasped, there ought to be money and workers forthcoming to carry it on.

The aim of this and the preceding chapters has been to suggest the lines along which modern science is leading us in psychology. We are gradually gaining sufficient knowledge of the mind to be able to give practical hints for its better conduct. In respect of this practical guidance psychology is behind physiology. More is known of the laws of physical than of mental health. We all understand the importance of fresh air, sunshine, exercise, simple food, and sleep. We are foolish if we disregard this knowledge, or ignore the aches and pains which give warning of an approaching illness ; we are equally foolish if, in the mental sphere, we leave to chance or " nature " what is really within our own power.

Nature might have been a good guide in the days when man's life was as simple as that of the highest animals. The vast development of material civilization has left man's

innate endowment far behind. " Nature " is as incapable
of leading a man to catch the right train in the morning,
as it is of making roses take root in the asphalt of Piccadilly.
We must study our own minds and give them all the help
that science can afford. To reject this help on the ground
that it is interfering with " nature " is to be as silly as the
man who rejected " Daylight Saving " on the ground that
it was interfering with " God's time ".

FOR DISCUSSION

1.—From the point of view of schools, what advantages have
Intelligence Tests over the ordinary examinations ?
2.—Go through a set of tests, e.g., the Otis or Northumberland tests,
and discover what are the mental qualities necessary for success
in them.
3.—For your own satisfaction make a list of your chief interests, and
state how you would attempt to find satisfaction for them in a
new town in which you had got work.
4.—Give an account of the formation of a friendship. Mention the
stages of development, and suggest means of maintaining it in
the future.

BOOKS

WILLIAM JAMES, " What makes a Life Significant ", in *Talks to Teachers*.
C. S. MYERS, *Present Day Applications of Psychology*. A little book
giving an account of psychology in industry and elsewhere.
CYRIL BURT, [1]*Mental and Scholastic Tests ; Handbook of Tests for Use in Schools*.
P. B. BALLARD, *Mental Tests ; Group Tests of Intelligence ; The New Examiner*.
Psychological Tests of Educable Capacity. Report of a Committee.
H.M. Stationery Office.
ARISTOTLE, *Nicomachean Ethics*, Bks. VIII and IX. A discussion on
Friendship.
Institute of Industrial Psychology. Reports.

---

[1] For advanced students.

ESSAY QUESTIONS

1.—Show in what ways instinct plays a part in mental development. Illustrate your answer by reference to the development of one of the following instincts : (a) self-preservation ; (b) curiosity ; (c) pugnacity.

2.—We cannot get rid of drudgery from school work, but we can at least invest that drudgery with meaning. Discuss this in reference to a particular class.

3.—Describe briefly any experiment you have seen in school which had for its object the development of *esprit de corps* among the children by the introduction of group competition in one form or another. Give your views as to the probable result on the children.

4.—Distinguish between suggestion and auto-suggestion, giving examples from child life of the working of each.

5.—By what means can good taste be inculcated in schools ?

6.—Study the play of any child you know, and show how that play is helping in his development.

7.—How would you discover whether a class of children was really attentive ? What steps would you take to deal with habitual inattention ?

8.—The ultimate aim of education is the training of the will. Do you accept this statement ? In what ways can a teacher facilitate the development of the will of the child ?

9.—What do you understand by sense training ? In what ways is it possible to develop sense perception, either in the infant school or with children who have passed beyond the infant stage ?

10.—What are the best ways of helping children to remember what they are taught ? Illustrate from some particular subject.

11.—In ordinary thought processes what part is played by visual imagery ? How does a recognition of this association help the teacher ?

12.—How far does imagination depend on memory ? Refer in your answer to older and younger children.

13.—At one stage in their development many children seem to prefer make-believe to reality. How far is this tendency to be encouraged, and what opportunities does it offer to the teacher ?

14.—Little children cannot reason. Is this true ? Give your own observations, stating the age of the children you have in mind.

ESSAY QUESTIONS

15.—What distinction is there between : (*a*) reasoning ; (*b*) following a train of rational thought as set out by a teacher ? Illustrate from any school subject the opportunities for (*a*).

16.—The primary aim of the school is to cultivate in its pupils the power of intelligent, ordered, and sustained effort. Discuss.

17.—Neatness, order and accuracy are matters of habit and discipline. Discuss this.

18.—How far and by what means can natural ability, as distinguished from the effects of teaching, be discovered in children ? How far should this ability be relied on as a basis for school classification ?

19.—What effects good and bad in teaching have followed from the assumption that there is an average child ?

20.—What considerations have led teachers to emphasize freedom rather than repression in their dealing with children in school ?

21.—Estimate the value of a system of rewards as (*a*) a stimulus to good work ; (*b*) as an aid to discipline.

22.—Looking back on your own schooldays what do you think were the results of encouragement or severity ?

23.—" If a teacher has secured the attention of the class he has all he needs." Discuss this and the best means of securing attention.

BIBLIOGRAPHY

Books by authors marked by a * are of more importance
than others.

LASCELLES ABERCROMBIE, *Theory of Poetry.*
*JOHN ADAMS, *Herbartian Psychology.*
*J. W. ADAMSON, *Short History of Education.*
A ADLER, *Individual Psychology.*
LEONID ANDREIEV, *The Seven that were Hanged.*
ARISTOTLE, *Nicomachean Ethics.*
   Poetics.
" ASTERISK ", *Gone Native.*
*W. C. BAGLEY, *Educative Process.*
*P. B. BALLARD, *Mental Tests.*
   Group Tests of Intelligence.
   New Examiner.
*C. BAUDOUIN, *Studies in Psycho-Analysis.*
MARK BENNY, *Low Company.*
*H. BERGSON, *Matter and Memory.*
*C. BIRCHENOUGH, *History of Elementary Education in England.*
JACK BLACK, *You Can't Win.*
A. BLACKWOOD, *Episodes before Thirty.*
G. LE BON, *The Crowd.*
W. A. BONE, *Service of the Hand in School.*
P. BOVET, *Fighting Instinct.*
G. F. BRADBY, *The Chronicles of Dawnhope.*
   Saga of Burnt Njal.
*C. BURT, *The Young Delinquent.*
   Mental and Scholastic Tests.
   Handbook of Tests.
   A Study in Vocational Guidance.
W. B. CANNON, *Bodily Changes in Fear, Hunger, Pain and Rage.*
G. D. H. COLE, *Labour in the Commonwealth.*
   Guild Socialism Restated.
*H. CALDWELL COOK, *The Playway.*
C. R. M. F. CRUTTWELL, *History of Peaceful Change in the Modern
World.*
C. DARWIN, *The Expression of the Emotions.*
DAY, *Sandford and Merton.*
E. M. DELAFIELD, *The War Workers.*

BIBLIOGRAPHY

*JOHN DEWEY, *Educational Essays.*
   How we Think.
G. B. DIBBLEE, *The Newspaper.*
DOSTOEFFSKI, *The House of the Dead.*
   The Possessed.
FISKE, *Witchcraft in Salem Village.*
FORESTER, *The General.*
*S. FREUD, *Interpretation of Dreams.*
ROGER FRY, *Art and Design.*
J. GALSWORTHY, *Loyalties.*
   Skin Game.
   Forsyte Saga.
*F. GALTON, *Inquiries into Human Faculty.*
*G. H. GREEN, *Psycho-Analysis in the Class-room.*
R. GRIFFITH, *Imagination in Early Childhood.*
K. GROOS, *Play of Man.*
RIDER HAGGARD, *Nada the Lily.*
T. HARDY, *Jude the Obscure.*
*B. HART, *The Psychology of Insanity.*
*HODGSON BURNETT, *The Secret Garden.*
*ALDOUS HUXLEY, *Brave New World.*
SUSAN ISAACS, *Social Development in Young Children.*
WILLIAM JAMES, *Text-book of Psychology.*
   Talks to Teachers, passim.
   Memories and Studies.
RICHARD JEFFERIES, *Bevis, a Boy.*
E. H. JONES, *Road to Endor.*
*C. G. JUNG, *Studies in Word Association.*
   Psychology of the Unconscious.
M. W. KEATINGE, *Suggestion in Education.*
MARGARET KENNEDY, *The Constant Nymph.*
*C. W. KIMMINS, *Children's Dreams.*
MELANIE KLEIN, *Psycho-Analysis of Children.*
W. KOEHLER, *Gestalt Psychology.*
PRINCE KROPOTKIN, *Fields, Factories and Workshops.*
EMILE LAUVRIÈRE, *La Vie d'Edgar A. Poe.*
   Laxdael Saga.
VERNON LEE, *The Beautiful.*
JACK LONDON, *Before Adam.*
   White Fang.
J. W. MARRIOTT, *Exercises in Thinking and Expression.*
J. MASEFIELD, *The Faithful.*
A. MAUROIS, *Ariel.*
J. S. MILL, *Utilitarianism.*
   Logic.
A. A. MILNE, *Peace with Honour.*
*P. MONROE, *Text-book in the History of Education.*
*M. MONTESSORI, *The Montessori Method.*
*C. S. MYERS, *Present-day Applications of Psychology.*
F. H. W. MYERS, *Human Personality and its Survival of Bodily Death.*

BIBLIOGRAPHY

Rose Macaulay, *Dangerous Ages.*
J. MacCunn, *Making of Character.*
W. McDougall, *Group Mind.*
            Social Psychology.
            Outline of Psychology.
            Body and Mind.
            Character and the Conduct of Life.
*M. Nicoll, *Dream Psychology.*
Harold Nicolson, *Tennyson.*
*T. P. Nunn, *Education, Its Data and First Principles.*
Osty, *Supernormal Faculties in Man.*
John Paris, *Kimono.*
Helen Parkhurst, *Dalton Plan.*
*T. H. Pear, *Remembering and Forgetting.*
Peckham, *Wasps, Social and Solitary.*
Plato, *Republic.*
*Morton Prince, *Dissociation of a Personality*
            The Unconscious.
Psychological Tests of Educable Capacity. H.M. Stationery Office.
Lord Redesdale, *Tales of Old Japan.*
A. I. Richards, *Hunger and Work in a Savage Tribe.*
I. A. Richards, *Principles of Criticism.*
*W. H. R. Rivers, *Instinct and the Unconscious.*
            Conflict and Dream.
            Psychology and Politics.
Sax Rohmer, *The Romance of Sorcery.*
Bertrand Russell, *Which Way to Peace.*
R. R. Rusk, *Experimental Education.*
M. E. Sadler, *Moral Instruction and Training in Schools.*
F. C. S. Schiller, *Doris Fischer Case.*
K. de Schweinitz, *How a Baby is Born.*
A. F. Shand, *Foundations of Character.*
Mrs. Sherwood, *History of the Fairchild Family.*
A. Sidgwick, *Elementary Logic.*
May Sinclair, *Life and Death of Harriett Freen.*
*Henrietta Brown Smith, *The Child under Eight.*
G. Elliot Smith, *Human History.*
*C. E. Spearman, *Nature of Intelligence.*
J. Steinbeck, *Maria Spiridonova.*
*G. F. Stout, *Manual of Psychology.*
            Analytic Psychology.
*H. Sturt, *Principles of Understanding.*
J. Swift, *Fable of Bee and Spider.*
            Battle of Books.
Tacitus, *Annals.*
Tarde, *The Laws of Imitation.*
R. H. Tawney, *Acquisitive Society.*
F. W. Taylor, *Scientific Management.*
Ordway Teed, *Instincts in Industry.*
G. Thomson, *Instinct, Intelligence and Character.*
G. L. Thorndike, *Educational Psychology.*

BIBLIOGRAPHY

A. TROLLOPE, *Autobiography.*
TROTSKI, *My Life.*
TRAVEN, *The Death Ship.*
W. TROTTER, *Instincts of the Herd in War and Peace.*
*GRAHAM WALLAS, *Our Social Heritage.*
　　　　　　　Great Society.
　　　　　　　Human Nature in Politics.
HUGH WALPOLE, *Mr. Perrin and Mr. Traill.*
FRANCIS WARD, *Animal Life under Water.*
M. J. WATT, *Economy and Training of Memory.*
ISAAC WATTS, *Hymns and Moral Poems.*
*A. K. WHITE and A. MACBEATH, *The Moral Self.*
FRANCIS WILLIAMS, *Plan for Peace.*
W. B. YEATS, *The King's Threshold.*

INDEX

Abilities, general, 242
— — graph exhibiting, 242
— — and special, relation between, 245, 246
— special, 242
— — anxiety to teachers caused
by children with, 243
— — graph exhibiting, 242
Abnormality, human, study of,
detailed, 7
Abstract objects, sentiments
formed for, 121
Academic work replaced by constructional in one type of
children, 95
Accuracy, love of, 238
— value of, needs teaching to
children, 238
Acquisition, 99
— books for consultation, 103
— sporadic, appearance among
animals, 99
Acquisitive tendency, explanation for, 99, 100
— — first reason for organization of, 100
— — in children, 99
Action, attention the precursor
of, 170
— habitual, proceeding without
thought, 213
Actions follow emotions, 105
— led to by habits, adjusted to
particular circumstances,
237
— not " right " and " wrong,"
psychologically, 5
Activities, human, purposeful-
ness of, 149
Activity in children, manifestation of, 291, 292

Activity instinctive, 22
— — books for consultation, 34
— — questions for discussion,
34
— mechanical versus purposive,
9
— — books for consultation, 21
— — questions for discussion,
20
— natural, not an incentive for
full work required, 143
— natural state of children and
most adults, 141
— progressive manifestation of,
in children, 141, 142
— pursuit under full compulsion, disadvantages of,
141
— two principal impulses for,
142
Actor, the, purposes denied by,
examples of, 17
Addition of figures, practice of,
234
Adjustment, disorders of, 265
— — — books for consultation,
275, 276
— — — questions for discussion, 275
Admiration, imitation due to,
how illustrated, 48
Adolescence, in relation to religious principles, 79
— interest in politics developing towards end of, 80
Adolescents, sexual anxiety in,
81
Adults, activity natural state of
majority of, 141
— aims years distant worked for
by, 16, 17

INDEX